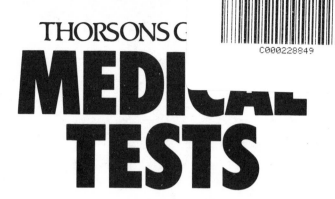

THORSONS C

MEDICAL
TESTS

C000228849

Joanna Trevelyan is a writer specializing in health issues and is currently Features Editor for *Nursing Times*.

Dr David Dowson has been a GP for 15 years and is now a full-time partner at the Centre for the Study of Complementary Medicine in Southampton. He has a particular interest in environmental medicine.

Ruth West is an experienced researcher into alternative medicine.

THORSONS GUIDE TO
MEDICAL TESTS

The complete handbook of diagnostic
and preventive tests

Joanna Trevelyan & Dr David Dowson
with Ruth West

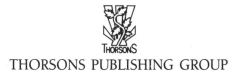

THORSONS PUBLISHING GROUP

First published 1989

British Library Cataloguing in Publication Data

Trevelyan, Joanna E. (Joanna Elanwy)
Thorsons guide to medical tests.
1. Medicine. Diagnosis
I. Title II. Dowson, David III. West, Ruth, *1948-*
616.07'5

ISBN 0-7225-1503-0

Published by Thorsons Publishers Limited,
Wellingborough, Northamptonshire, NN8 2RQ, England

Printed in Great Britain by Woolnough Bookbinding Limited,
Irthlingborough, Northamptonshire
Typeset by MJL Limited, Hitchin, Hertfordshire

1 3 5 7 9 10 8 6 4 2

CONTENTS

Picture Credits

Photographs: Bruce Coleman pages 21 and 25; Dr Jane Chomet page 213; Dan McCoy from Rainbow page 178; Bill Pierce from Rainbow page 36; Science Photo Library pages 31, 33, 74 and 203; John Watney pages 28 and 139.

Line illustrations by Jane Bottomley.

Chapter 1

INTRODUCTION

While consumers are now more aware of the fallibility of many treatments by our medical profession, medical testing still enjoys a high degree of trust from the public. We assume that the battery of tests we are so often subjected to are, first and foremost, necessary. We also believe that they will accurately diagnose what is wrong, or screen successfully for hidden problems. The fact is that few tests reach this ideal, and despite an enormous increase in the numbers performed, there has been no commensurate increase in accurate diagnosis or screening. There can also be real dangers associated with many medical tests, from the technique itself, and from human error or improper use.

The aim of this book is to open up medical testing to general discussion, in the hope that, with better informed consumers, testing will undergo critical evaluation so that fewer unnecessary, sometimes dangerous — not to mention expensive — tests will be performed.

WHY ARE TESTS USED?

One of the main purposes of this book is to clarify the gap between what medical tests are expected and assumed to do, and their actual value in the care of patients, in the hope that patients can then use this knowledge to demand their proper use.

Ostensibly, tests are designed to assist the clinical judgement of the doctor — not, it must be emphasized, to take its place — by:

- screening for the presence of disease

- confirming a diagnosis of disease

7

- unearthing possible alternative diagnoses

- monitoring the progress of treatment

- checking that a diagnosis is correct

- providing prognostic information

HOW NECESSARY ARE MEDICAL TESTS?

A two-year study of out-patients at a certain district hospital showed that of the three basic clinical methods — history, examination and investigation — the history was the most important factor in both diagnosis and management in cardiovascular, neurological, respiratory, urinary and other miscellaneous problems, and decided 56% of all diagnoses and 46% of all management. Examination findings were of limited value, accounting for only 17% of diagnostic and 17% of management decisions overall. No matter what the disorder was shown to be, blood and urine tests were almost worthless, contributing to less than 1% of diagnoses.

There is, in fact, quite widespread agreement within the medical profession that far too many unnecessary tests are performed, many of them as routine. The problem which has arisen is that there is no way of reducing their number without interfering with the doctor's right to exercise his clinical judgement whether and when tests are needed. For a variety of reasons, that judgement is all too often unsound.

The problem may lie in the training of doctors, who are just not taught the skills necessary to interpret the results of the increasingly complex and large range of tests available, but who are also tempted more and more to rely on tests because they are supposed to be more 'scientific' than the use of history-taking and personal judgement. Or the problem may lie in specialization: specialists, there is evidence to show, often order more tests, even though this leads to no difference in clinical outcome.

However, the blame cannot be laid entirely at the doctor's door. Other causes have been traced: to automation in laboratories, so that it is as easy to perform ten tests as one; to hospital procedure, so that a whole batch of routine, non-discretionary tests are carried out on admission; to the state of the art, which means that there is a genuine mismatch between the sophistication of some modern diagnostic tests and the use to which the knowledge they give can be put: they are in advance of the treatment for the disease. The list goes on. Dr A H W Wahba, of the World Health Organization's 'Health Care Technology Programme' has assembled 36 reasons for carrying out medical tests. Sadly, few are strictly related to the needs and interests of the patients concerned.

Reasons for carrying out medical tests

1 **Related to physicians and health care personnel:**
- Confirmation of a clinical opinion
- Diagnosis (predictive or current)
- Monitoring
- Prognosis
- Routine check-up
- Screening
- Unavailability of a previous result
- Peer pressure
- Physician and other staff insecurity and reassurance
- Completion of data base
- Over-specialization
- Research
- Curiosity
- Frustration
- Personal profit
- Establishing a base line
- Education (personal, other staff, students)
- Tradition
- Habit

2 Related to technology

- Questionable accuracy of a previous result
- Pressure from recent publications, industry, promotion, conferences, seminars
- Ease and simplicity of performance
- Inexpensive procedure
- Ready availability
- Lack of information on advantages, limitations, appropriateness
- Provision of annotated and printed result

3 Related to patients

- Patient/family pressure
- Patient/family reassurance
- Pleasing particular types of patients
- Buying time
- Showing that 'something' is done

4 Related to administration

- Documentation and completion of file
- Hospital profit
- Hospital or national policies and requirements (on admission, preoperative, follow-up, predischarge)
- Legal requirement
- Medico-legal need

HOW ARE THE TESTS SELECTED?

A doctor is given guidance in his selection of tests by information on their 'operating characteristics'; that is, their accuracy as measured by:

- their ability to exclude the presence of a disease because of their level of *sensitivity* — that is, how often they are positive in patients with the disease being tested for; and

- their ability to confirm the presence of a disease because of their *specificity*, which indicates how often the tests are negative in those without the disease in question

Tests rarely combine both sensitivity and specificity — so few can be used to both exclude the likelihood of a certain disease and confirm its presence. It is also important to realize that tests do not need to be 100% accurate — in terms of specificity or sensitivity — in order to be of use. This means that you may well be given a test that is only 80% accurate; that is, that gives a false result in 20 out of every 100 cases. Some widely used tests have only a 50% accuracy; so, for example, 15 out of 31 tests given to patients suffering from rheumatoid arthritis were eliminated prior to the commencement of a recent study on the grounds that more than 50% of the results of these tests were 'within the reference range for healthy controls'.

It is the doctor's task to calculate the post-test probability of the likelihood of the disease, taking into account the pre-test likelihood of the disease being present and a test's sensitivity and/or specificity — or sometimes what is known as the 'likelihood ratio' used to evaluate a test's performance. And there are further considerations and judgements to be made in selecting and evaluating the results of a test. One of these is just how significant a test is. It may be highly accurate — yet show a positive or abnormal result in a multitude of different diseases. A second is whether the laboratory or clinic carrying out the test is competently run (are the technicians sufficiently trained and reliable?); a third, whether the machinery is in good working order; a fourth is knowing what might bias the results of a test, such as drugs the patient may be taking, his or her diet, and so on. All the checks are essential if patients are to be spared needless anxiety, and perhaps even unnecessary treatment as a consequence of test results.

On the whole, medical tests have not yet been critically evaluated to determine how necessary they are — let alone how safe they are — in medical practice.

HOW ARE NEW TESTS INTRODUCED?

The worrying fact is that even the sanctioned way of establishing a test — by clinical controlled trial — is not necessary for a test to become an accepted part of practice; so there are many tests that have been in use for years, without anyone specifically evaluating them.

The case of amniocentesis, a routine test undergone by about 20,000 pregnant women a year in England to diagnose such conditions as spina bifida and Down's syndrome, is salutary. But it was around for at least 15 years before, in 1986, any research results of the test were published. And these first results suggested some risk that the test disrupted foetal lung development. It is going to take further studies — with perhaps further risk for new-born babies — to find out whether the test may cause any long-term effects on lung function.

The lack of any established system responsible for research and dissemination of results of new medical tests leaves room for a variety of extraneous influences, such as the enthusiasm of those employing and believing in the test, or pressure of consumer demand.

Two further problems regarding the evaluation of new tests need mentioning. The first is that information about tests as they come into use takes a long time before it is accepted into the medical literature, and so disseminated. By the time this has occurred, the test, because of the rapid developments taking place in modern technological medicine, has often become obsolete. But the second and more important problem lies with our present system — or rather lack of system — of controls for medical technology. Until there is one body with the responsibility for seeing that the necessary research is done before any new test is introduced — which will require statutory changes — there will always be ways of getting unevaluated new tests accepted and used.

IS CHANGE POSSIBLE?

Enough people and organizations have voiced their concern, expressed their ideas — and had them published — that it now seems there is a consensus that something must be done. But what? And how? The World Health Organization has taken a lead. Through its global programme, 'Coming to Terms with Health

Technology', it aims to set up channels of communication to provide information, advice and expertise to decision-makers. For it believes that 'it is not necessarily true that there is insufficient money — but it is true that the available resources are not wisely spent'.

One way of remedying this was suggested at a 1987 King's Fund forum on the subject of screening for pregnant women. The discussion highlighted the need for cost benefit analysis of tests that went beyond monetary information on costs and savings to include social and clinical measures; benefits such as 'the provision of authoritative information, relief from uncertainty, support during a period of crisis. . .'

The worrying delays while confirmatory tests are conducted, the distress that may result from false positive results, and the illusory reassurance given by false negative results — these all have their price tag, even if it is not paid for by the NHS, but some other service at some later date, which should be taken into account when decisions are made on the allocation of health service budgets.

Such information, of course, should also be available to those who select and use medical tests: doctors. Other recommendations cover their training at both undergraduate and postgraduate levels. This, it is widely agreed, must now provide adequate instruction on the appropriate use and interpretation of test results: and, it has been suggested, should include learning to become familiar with the latest computer-based systems in order to keep up to date with the strides being made in technological medicine.

However, this alone may be insufficient. Rationing of tests may be far more useful; but what is really needed is research into 'the behaviour modification' of doctors, and in particular how they can be made to perceive people as human beings, possessing emotions and responding to their environment, and not just complex machines. In the meantime, protocols controlling requests for tests and the redesigning of test forms would serve a useful purpose in curtailing those which are unnecessary.

The choice is becoming clear. To keep with a medical service committed to the servicing and repair of complicated human machines at a horrifyingly high cost, or to move towards a wider perspective, that is informed by a consideration of the human, psycho-social factors in disease, and has as its goal the promotion of health over the treatment or prevention of disease. Although the considerations of such a perspective lie beyond the scope of this book it guides its purpose. And, who knows? Such a change in attitude may have as much effect on the way in which medical tests are used as enforced legislation.

Chapter 2

DIAGNOSTIC TESTS

Diagnosis is the process of determining the nature of a disorder. To do so, doctors use information from:

- the patient's 'signs' — indications of a disorder observed by the doctor, but not apparent to the patient.

- the patient's 'symptoms' — indications of a disorder noticed by the patient.

- the medical background of the patient and his/her family.

- the results of diagnostic tests.

The first three of these sources of information constitute history and can provide an accurate diagnosis in more than 80% of patients. Laboratory test results, on the other hand, have been shown to change the diagnosis in only 10% of cases. One study reported that routine blood and urine tests contributed to less than 1% of all diagnoses. Tests results should therefore only play a support role in diagnosis and never be the sole diagnostic tool employed.

Rather worryingly it has been estimated that more than 50 per cent of all tests ordered are less than 80% accurate. A US Government study concluded that more than one out of every seven test results were wrong or unreliable. All this adds up to a lot of unnecessary anxiety and treatment for the patient. Having to undergo unnecessary testing is not simply a waste of time and money. It can be a health hazard: continued exposure to invasive procedures can weaken your body and leave you open to infection — in effect, doctor induced. If this was not enough, there is often disagreement among doctors about the interpretation of a test result. In a study of doctors' reading of X-rays, more than 70% of reports contained disagreements among experienced radiologists. Whatever the test, it is thought that between 10 and 20% of doctors will miss an important test finding. Surprisingly, patients still think medical tests are infallible.

So how are medical tests evaluated? Usually the following parameters are assessed:

Sensitivity: how often the test shows a positive result when in fact more than one disease is present.

Specificity: how often the test shows a negative result when an individual does not have the condition being tested for.

(The combined percentage values of sensitivity and specificity provide a reasonable indication of a test's accuracy).

Predictive value: the probability of the existence of a disease should a medical test show the positive result for that disease.

Significance: this refers to how precise a test is for a particular disease. The most significant test will be one that is positive only for one condition, but no such tests are currently available. Understanding a test's significance is vital in making decisions about when a certain test should be performed, and in interpreting the results. Unfortunately, fewer than 5% of doctors in a leading medical centre in the US were found to be able to correctly apply the concept of predictive value.

Test results can be affected by a number of things:

- the presence of certain medications in the patient

- certain foods, routine activities, attitudes (for example, fear and stress distort the hormone balance)

- physical factors such as sex, age, height and weight

- pregnancy

- the presence of other medical conditions

Ascertain from your doctor what might affect your test result. Tell him/her if you have any allergies to food or medication, remind him/her of anything which might effect the procedure — being diabetic or pregnant, for example. Ask him/her if there is anything you should do, or avoid, prior to the test.

A positive result does not necessarily mean you have the disease in question — the range of normal values may not be appropriate to you; the test result may be inaccurate, or you may have done or eaten something that affected the result. Ask for the test to be repeated until a consistent result is obtained.

In order to ensure you are getting the best and most appropriate tests available there are some basic questions to ask your doctor before agreeing to any procedure:

- **Why do you need the test? What information will it give that is not already available?**

- **What is it supposed to detect?**

- **How accurate is it?**

- **What risks are there?**

- **Is there a less dangerous, less invasive alternative?**

- **What will happen in the test?**

- **When will the results be available, and what will a positive result mean to you?**

Only when you are satisfied with the answers should you go ahead. Doctors are now more willing to answer questions, but they do not have to. The law only requires that a patient be given 'information suitable to his education and intelligence to permit him to assess fairly the proposed examination or treatment'. The doctor, not the patient, decides what is 'suitable'. Many hospitals still have consent forms for 'whatever may be necessary' that patients are asked to sign on admission. However, since the patient in many cases cannot be properly aware of what he is consenting to, such consent has no legal validity.

Having certain tests may affect your ability to undertake other tests, or make it necessary to avoid certain things, so always tell all those involved with your case that you have had a test. After the test, chase up your results and ask to have them fully explained to you. Twenty five to fifty per cent of all abnormal results reported are not followed up by the doctor. It is your body and your life — ignoring a test result could prove fatal.

CLINICAL LABORATORY TESTS

URINE TESTS

Urinalysis is a useful test of the general health of the body. It is also a specific measure of kidney function and pregnancy. Overall, it is considered 90% accurate.

Routine urinalysis can be performed in a doctor's surgery or clinic and on admission to a hospital. Testing for specific compounds in the urine is also performed in the emergency room, intensive care, and on the ward of the hospital.

Urine can be collected as a random specimen, an early morning specimen or as a timed collection. It is important that you are given clear, unambiguous instructions because if the procedure is not followed exactly, you may invalidate the test results.

The chemical composition of a urine specimen can be determined by dipping a multi-chemically coated paper in the urine. This allows up to ten separate urine examinations to be performed simultaneously. Urine can also be examined microscopically and cultured.

STOOLS TESTS

Stools are collected from a hospital patient in a bedpan. As an outpatient you will be given a glass jar. You should not urinate into the bedpan or jar at the time of stool collection and it is essential that all faeces are collected. The stools will be examined for their appearance and may be taken for microscopic examination or culture.

BLOOD TESTS

These include:

Blood chemistry tests of substances dissolved in the blood fluid.

Hematologic tests of the size, shape and other characteristics of the blood cells themselves.

Serologic tests of the blood for antibodies, immune complexes, antigen-antibody reactions.

Groups of tests often ordered together include: complete blood count; analysis of electrolytes; liver function tests and thyroid function tests.

A small number of blood tests can be carried out by your GP in his surgery, but usually blood samples are sent to laboratories for testing. Blood tests can be done at home, hospital or a clinic, and may be taken by a doctor, nurse or a technician. Certain blood tests are also amenable to self testing particularly those related to the monitoring of a diabetic condition (see Chapter 4).

There are three ways of obtaining a blood sample:

VENEPUNCTURE

As veins are more accessible, being closer to the skin, this is the most common method of sampling. A tourniquet is wrapped tightly around your upper arm to stop the flow of blood through the veins, and you may be asked to open and close your hand or squeeze a cylinder-shaped object. This makes the veins bulge beneath the skin, and therefore easier to insert a needle. The skin is cleaned and a needle inserted. The blood then flows into the syringe or container. More than one sample can be taken while the needle is in place. When the needle is withdrawn, the tourniquet is removed and a dressing is placed over the puncture site. You will be asked to maintain pressure on the dressing for a few minutes to help stop the bleeding — this also prevents bruising. A plaster or small bandage will then be applied.

The pain and discomfort you experience depends on the skill of the person doing the test. It is also easier to perform on some people than others — depending on the accessibility of the veins in the arm and even on toughness of the skin. Do mention if there have been any previous problems with blood tests, and if you usually feel faint while having a blood test, ask to lie down during the collection. Sterile disposable needles are always used, so there is no risk of infection.

FINGER STICK

A drop or two of blood is taken from a finger, earlobe, or heel (in babies) by lancing the skin with a tiny sterile needle. The blood is then put on specially prepared strips of paper for testing.

ARTERIAL STICK

A few tests require a sample of blood from an artery. This is usually taken from inside of the wrist, or sometimes the groin. You sit with your arm extended and your wrist on a pillow. The doctor rotates your hand back and forth while feeling your pulse. The wrist is cleansed and you may have a small amount of local anaesthetic injected before the needle is inserted into the artery. Insertion is more painful than with a venepuncture because the arteries are deeper and have more nerves. After the needle is removed the puncture will be bandaged and firm pressure applied for at least five minutes.

CEREBROSPINAL FLUID TESTS

Cerebrospinal fluid is normally collected by lumbar puncture. It is usually performed in hospital by a physician, sometimes with an assistant. Before the test, tell your doctor if you have any allergies to medications or anaesthetics, if you are taking medication or if you have bleeding problems. You may be asked to sign a consent form so be sure you are satisfied with the information you have been given. The doctor will give you a neurologic examination to check for signs of increased pressure to your brain — it is dangerous to perform the test if there is. You will need to empty your bowels and bladder before the procedure is carried out. You will either be asked to sit, bending slightly forward, or to lie on your side with knees raised in the foetal position. The

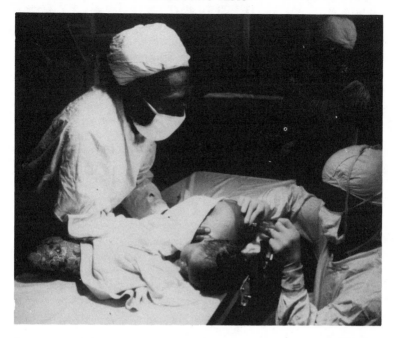

Figure 1. Two doctors carrying out a lumbar puncture on a small baby.

assistant may help you maintain your position, and should reassure you as to what is happening. A small needle is placed in the back, between the lumbar (lower back) vertebrae, and the fluid is withdrawn. Collection takes between ten and 20 minutes.

The test should not be painful as a local anaesthetic is usually used, although some people find the positions rather uncomfortable to maintain. After the test you will be asked to lie flat in bed for a few hours (up to 24) in order to reduce the chance of a headache. Some doctors encourage you to drink fluids to help prevent headaches and other side effects — they should provide you with a straw while lying down! The risks include haemorrhage in the area of needle penetration, especially if the needle is improperly placed or if you move. Approximately one out of every 1000 patients who undergoes cerebrospinal fluid testing suffers nerve paralysis, although in most cases the paralysis is reversible. Check when your results will be ready as this can vary. If your spinal fluid appears abnormal on extraction, you will be closely observed and a series of brief neurological tests may be performed periodically for the first few hours after the test.

SPUTUM TESTS

Evaluation of sputum specimens is useful in the diagnosis of diseases of the lower respiratory tract. Sputum is the mucus that is coughed up from the respiratory tract, mixed with a small amount of saliva. In order to collect a sample, you should cough deeply and the material should come from the lungs. Usually the first-morning specimen is requested. In order to reduce contamination by the normal flora of the mouth, the mouth should be rinsed out before coughing. The test is usually done in hospital, and the specimen is delivered to the laboratory immediately for microscopic examination and/or culture. The results will be available in a few days, although cultures for TB may take up to six weeks, so check beforehand.

TESTS USING OTHER BODILY SECRETIONS

AMNIOTIC FLUID ANALYSES

See Chapter 5 p 175.

DRAINING WOUNDS FOR ANAEROBIC INFECTIONS

Samples are removed using a sterile swab for microscopic examination and/or culture. This may be painful depending on where the sample is being removed from.

GASTRIC SAMPLING

This is performed in hospital where you will first be asked to fast for at least 12 hours. A tube is then passed through the nose or mouth into the stomach and gastric fluid withdrawn by suction for one hour. An injection of histamine may be given to stimulate maximal acid production, in which case the gastric fluid is tested again one hour later. An alternative, although less accurate, test is to swallow a dye, after which the colour of the urine is noted.

There are virtually no risks in the tube or dye method, although the insertion of the tube is clearly going to be uncomfortable.

SEMEN

See Chapter 7 p 227.

SWEAT

This is collected by using a drug that induces sweating. A gauze pad or filter paper containing the drug is placed on a cleansed forearm (or on the thigh or shoulder blade of small babies) and an electrode is placed over it and a constant current of 2 milli-amp applied for about five minutes. This may cause a tingling sensation. Then the electrode and gauze are removed and the arm cleansed and dried. A preweighed filter paper is then applied to the forearm and covered by plastic secured with tape. After 30 minutes, the filter paper is removed and sent immediately to the laboratory for analysis. This test is most commonly used as a diagnosis for cystic fibrosis.

CULTURES

The purpose of a culture is to isolate and identify the microbes that cause disease through infection. Since virtually every part of the body is subject to infection, the test is performed on many tissues, secretions, excretions and fluids. The sample will have been collected using techniques such as those described above, then placed in two or more containers, each containing a different medium (one to grow organisms in the presence of air and one to grow them without air). It usually takes between two and ten days for culture reports to be available. Cultures can be performed to

● **find the cause of an infection**

● **test the body's ability to fight off infection**

● test which particular antibiotic will be effective

● test which antibody would be the best to use on a particular infection.

All these tests are considered to be 95% accurate, although the results can be inconclusive — especially if the sample was inadequate. You should tell your doctor if you are on any antibiotics before a culture is performed. Depending on what bodily product is being cultured there may be certain things you should or should not do, for example, if it is a sputum culture you should drink as much fluid as possible as this keeps the membranes in your respiratory tract moist and will help you cough up the needed sample. So check what preparation, if any, is needed.

IMAGING TECHNIQUES

RADIOGRAPHY

Radiography is a technique for examining the body using a form of electromagnetic radiation — X-rays. It is used in the diagnosis of disorders where inspection from outside the body is insufficient. The X-rays are directed through the body to produce images on photographic plates or fluorescent screens (radiographs). Because there is a differential absorption of X-rays by different tissues, the resultant radiograph shows anatomical details of the part of the body examined. The denser the tissue, the whiter they will appear on the radiograph, whereas empty space appears black. In order to highlight a particular organ, a substance that shows up on X-rays is sometimes introduced into the body. These are called contrast materials, contrast media or dyes. You should be screened for any allergy to these beforehand.

Radiological procedures are performed on an in- or out-patient basis at the hospital. They should only be carried out by specially trained radiographers.

Before undergoing any radiological procedure you will be asked to take off certain clothing and jewellery. Depending on what is being examined, you will be required to assume various positions while sitting, standing, or lying supine on an X-ray table. The radi-

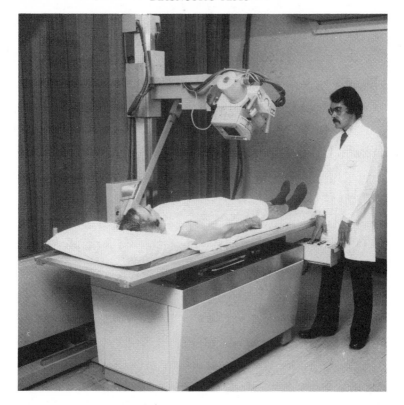

Figure 2. A patient undergoing X-ray tomography.

ographer should explain clearly what is expected of you before the X-ray is taken.

X-rays do bring certain risks with them:

- damage to living cells and tissue;

- damage to a developing foetus (so always notify your doctor if you might be pregnant);

- damage to sperm or egg cells in the testes or ovaries possibly resulting in sterility or defects in future children.

All such effects can take months and even years before manifesting themselves. Your personal risk from X-ray exposure depends on

- your age (children are more sensitive to X-ray damage)

- the area of the body being X-rayed (certain organs such as bone marrow are more sensitive than others), and

- the amount of radiation you have received in the past (as the effect is cumulative).

You should discuss with your doctor how these risks affect you to assess whether they outweigh potential benefits of the procedure. It is important to establish whether the test is really necessary, because many unnecessary X-rays are ordered every day, often as substitutes for thorough examination and history taking.

When the test involves only a simple X-ray picture, there is no pain or discomfort. When multiple X-rays are performed over a period of time, you may experience discomfort from lying or sitting on a hard table. Some of the additional procedures associated with radiography, such as barium meals or enemas can cause discomfort or embarrassment. The use of injected contrast material such as dyes to outline blood vessels for example, can cause a great deal of pain for days, if the injection of the dye misses the vein.

The results of most radiographic tests are essentially subjective, depending primarily on a doctor's interpretation. Unless the pathology is obvious, a radiologist can easily miss something important — a fracture, ulcer, or even a cancerous growth. For example, it is estimated from research that there is an error of 20 to 50% in the detection of cancers that are visible on X-rays. With an increase in the demand for X-rays there is a growing problem of lack of properly trained radiographers. This in turn leads to X-rays being undertaken and interpreted by inadequately trained personnel.

On average, radiography is only about 50% accurate, the inaccuracy resulting from

- poor technique in taking the X-ray pictures

- faulty equipment

- relatively untrained interpretation, and

- the subjective nature of the results.

ULTRASOUND

Ultrasound is a diagnostic technique that uses sound waves rather than X-rays to create an image of certain areas of the body. It is carried out by trained technicians or doctors in hospital either on a in- or out-patient basis.

High frequency sound waves (inaudible to us) are directed at the area of the body under examination using a transducer — a microphone like instrument that emits sounds and also detects the echo that comes from the body. The echoes are transmitted into an image or a graph on a screen. Before the transducer is applied, a coating of oil is applied to the skin to prevent any air from coming between the body and the instrument.

There may be some preparation necessary before undergoing the ultrasound, such as an enema if it is your abdomen that is being scanned. Your doctor should tell you what will be necessary. You should ask if there is anything, such as certain medications, that might affect the results. For example, ultrasound should not be performed on a woman fitted with an intra-uterine contraceptive device (IUD or coil).

For the test you will be asked to take off clothes and jewellery that cover the area to be examined and to lie on your back on an examining table, where the oil or gel will be applied. An ultrasound generally takes about 15 to 20 minutes and the only discomfort should be having to maintain a particular position for that length of time.

In order to measure moving objects in the body, such as the heart beat or the blood flowing through an artery, *Doppler Ultrasound* is used. Sound waves that are reflected back from moving objects show a change in frequency with changes in the speed of movement. For example, if the blood flow is rapid, the sound is high pitched, if blood flow is slow, a low pitched sound is produced. You may be asked not to smoke for a period of time before such a test, as nicotine can constrict the arteries.

Because ultrasound cannot travel through air and bone, it cannot be used in examinations of bones, the lungs or the brain. Some patients may also be difficult to scan — particularly if obese (thick layers of fat may block sound waves), or with unhealed incisions or large scars over the area to be studied.

There are no known risks to ultrasound, but it must be borne in mind that it was not so long ago that the medical profession thought X-rays were without risk. Various studies have shown ultrasound to be 80 to 90% accurate in detecting internal pathology. It is extremely valuable in outlining the foetus during pregnancy and helping to detect potential abnormalities. Accuracy problems have been attributed to the quality of interpretation: it is only as good as the technician and physician employing it.

NUCLEAR SCAN

Nuclear scanning, or radionucleotide organ imaging, is a diagnostic technique which outlines the size, shape, and exact location of an organ, chamber or duct within an organ. It can also measure organ function. Scans are used in the evaluation of patients with malignancies, and cardiovascular, abdominal, pulmonary, renal and thyroid disease.

A radioactive material (radioisotope or radionucleotide) is injected, ingested, or inhaled into the body, depending on the organ to be studied. The radionucleotide is composed of a chemical which 'homes in' on the organ to be examined. It can then be detected within the organ by rectilinear scanners or gamma cameras, both of which work on the same principle as the Geiger counter. Some radionucleotides concentrate on abnormal or dis-

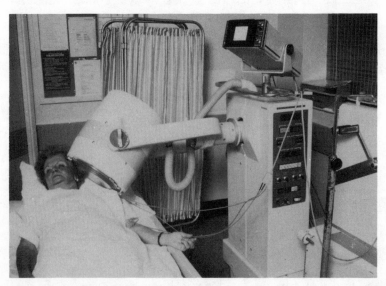

Figure 3. The equipment used for a nuclear scan.

eased tissue and form 'hot spots' on the scans. Others concentrate on normal tissue and avoid abnormal areas. Thus the abnormalities appear as areas of decreased radioactivity labelled 'cold spots'. The scans must be interpreted by a physician trained in nuclear medicine for an accurate evaluation to be made.

Nuclear scanning is always performed in hospital by specialists. It can be performed on an out-patient basis. The procedure varies according to the part of the body under investigation. Whatever the organ, you should tell your doctor if you are pregnant or breastfeeding.

Your doctor should tell you well in advance if any foods or liquid should be avoided prior to the test, or whether any medication or other medical procedure might interfere with the results. Before the test you will be asked to remove appropriate clothing and jewellery, and may be asked to empty your bladder. You will then be asked to lie on a table, above which is a large scanning camera. Some scans involve long waiting periods so it is a good idea to come prepared with magazines or books to while away the time. The actual scans may only take about five minutes, although a bone scan takes about an hour.

The scan is painless — bar the initial injection. To inject the radionucleotide, a tourniquet is placed on your arm or leg to make the vein more visible to inject into. Depending on the organ, you either have a wait until the tracer has distributed itself or the scanning camera will immediately be used to plot the movement of the tracer.

Before a bone scan you will be asked to drink four to six glasses of fluid to help clear your body of the radioactive material that is not picked up by the bone tissue. You will then have to empty your bladder before the test commences. For thyroid scans you will have been given a capsule or liquid containing a small amount of radioactive iodine and asked to swallow it six hours before the test is scheduled to begin. You may resume a normal diet one to two hours after swallowing the iodine.

You may have a series of pictures taken over a period of time, with perhaps an interval of an hour between each picture. It is important to establish with your doctor how long the whole procedure will take in order to estimate how long you are likely to be in hospital. For example, if you have a whole body scan (gallium scan), pictures will usually be taken at six hours, 24 hours, 48 hours and sometimes 72 hours after the injection. Also check when the results will be made available as this does vary. The amount of radioactivity in a radionucleotide is very small, and is eliminated from the body within a few days. The risks of this test are about the same as for X-ray procedures. For this reason they are not recommended for pregnant or breast-feeding women or young children. The scanning machines that are used to detect the radioactivity do not give off any radiation. As with any test you should weigh up the benefits and risks before undertaking the test.

COMPUTERIZED TOMOGRAPHY

This is a development of diagnostic radiology which provides a cross-sectional image of the organ or part of the body under examination. An extremely narrow X-ray beam is passed through a cross section of the body (or the brain) and is picked up by an electronic machine called a scintillator. The scintillator then feeds into a computer exactly what density of tissue the X-ray passed through. The computer then produces an image: high density tissue such as bone come out white in the picture, whereas liquids and air, which are of the lowest density, come out black. In between are all shades of gray, representing various organs and tissues. The images may be viewed on a TV screen or reproduced as photographs for permanent study.

There are two different forms of computerised tomography (CT): brain scanning and whole-body scanning. The machines used for each type of scanning are slightly different, but all require the patient to remain absolutely motionless for accurate results. For a CT scan you will be asked to lie on a table which is attached to the scanner. During the scan the table moves a small amount over a few seconds in order to position you for the next 'slice' or cross section. The X-ray camera and scintillator also rotate extremely rapidly around the body section being photographed so as to include everything in equal focus. If you move during the scan, the procedure will have to be repeated. Before you leave the scans may be checked, and if they are not adequate you may be asked to repeat them. The scan is not painful, but it can be uncomfortable to maintain the same position for several minutes at a time. If contrasting materials are used, there may be some discomfort when they are injected.

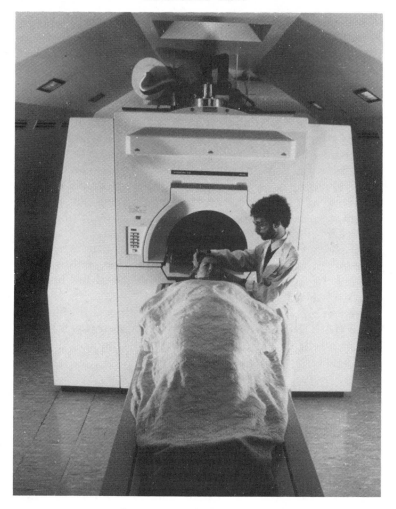

Figure 4. A person about to undergo a diagnostic scan using NMR (nuclear magnetic resonance) imaging.

CT scans have been shown to prevent unnecessary diagnostic and therapeutic surgery being performed and to substitute for many more invasive and potentially dangerous tests. There are fewer risks involved with CT than routine X-rays, but repeated CT scans will allow radiation to accumulate.

CT scanning is a very effective technique for diagnosing most forms of brain disease. However, there is a tendency for CT scans to produce false-negative tests. So a negative result should not

31

be considered absolute evidence of the absence of the disease. Total body scans are thought to be about 95% accurate.

THERMOGRAPHY

The human body gives off electromagnetic waves within the infra red spectrum. These waves are influenced by the temperature of your tissues. Irritated, infected tissue gives off more heat, and so does tissue that contains cancer. Radiation of heat can be measured and recorded. There are various different techniques of thermography, all of which are non-invasive and non-ionising. The patient is scanned in front of a detector which then transduces the radiant infra red energy (3 to 14 nm) into an electric signal for display on a cathode ray tube. The exam is conducted in an ambient temperature of 20 degrees celsius after cooling for 15 minutes. Under these conditions the surface of the breast is approximately 30 degrees celsius.

The trouble with thermography in detecting early cancers is that it yields too many false-positives and false-negatives so cannot be considered as an effective screening technique on its own.

MAGNETIC RESONANCE IMAGING

This is one of the latest techniques in diagnostic medicine. It can produce an image of the body far more revealing than any other imaging technique. It is also without the risks of X-ray and radionucleotide techniques — although it is too early to say if it is completely without risks. It is certainly painless. Unfortunately there are, to date, very few MRI scanners in British hospitals (less than 20).

Magnetic resonance imaging uses huge magnets and takes advantage of the fact that a large proportion of the human body is composed of water, which contains hydrogen atoms. When you put hydrogen atoms in a magnetic field and bombard them with radiowaves, they move into a high energy state. When the radiowaves are turned off, each atom will release the extra energy generated in the form of a faint radio signal. (Other atoms also react in a similar way and can be distinguished). A computer converts the signals into a picture according to the type and strength of the

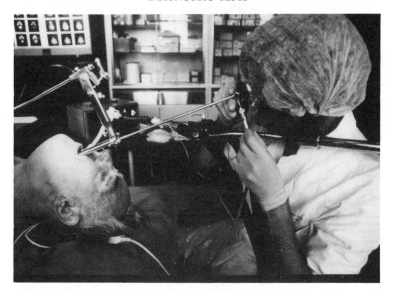

Figure 5. A doctor using a bronchoscope.

call sign. So a piece of fatty tissue with a lot of water will appear different from bone, which contains very little water.

In preparation for this test, you must remove all metal or metallic objects from your body since such objects may be attracted to the powerful magnet used in the procedure. If you have a pacemaker, artificial limb, or any other implanted or prosthetic medical device, discuss appropriate preparation and precautions with your doctor, because the magnetism is so powerful that it can send metallic objects flying. The test cannot be done on women with IUDs. After removing metal objects you will then be asked to lie on a table inside a cylindrical magnet. The table will be moved so that the part of your body to be examined lies in the centre of the magnet. It is important that you remain still while the test is in progress. You will feel nothing from the test which normally takes about 30 minutes.

The results are usually available in a couple of days.

TRANSILLUMINATION

This involves shining a very intense, cool light through the organ under investigation and noting the shadows it casts. This light

33

can be recorded on film. Light transmission is a helpful tool, but it is not very accurate when compared with X-ray mammography. It is used to differentiate cyst from solid mass in diagnosing breast disease. The patient is examined in a semi-darkened room with the light source under the breast as the physician palpates and compresses the breast to assure entire visualization of the chest wall. From available data, transillumination may be approaching the diagnostic accuracy of X-ray, but little has been done to assess its use as a screening method.

SCOPING PROCEDURES

Scoping procedures rely on a variety of viewing instruments which are used to look inside many organs and body spaces. These devices vary from simple magnifying lenses, to lighted telescopes, to extremely complex fibre optic viewing systems which can bend light rays so that the doctor can see around corners and obstacles and pinpoint the exact location of any pathology. All these instruments are usually equipped not only to allow for observation but also to

● **pump air into the cavity so as to extend the walls and make observation easier**

● **wash away anything that may obstruct the view (such as blood when looking for a bleeding ulcer)**

● **suction out suspected material for cytology tests, and**

● **take a biopsy specimen for testing.**

Photographs, even video pictures, can also be taken through some viewing instruments to offer a more permanent record of the inside view.

The actual procedure for scoping varies enormously depending what is to be viewed. Ask your doctor to explain exactly what will happen. Questions should include:

● **Will the test be done in hospital, with an overnight stay, or will it be performed on an out-patient basis?**

- What preparation will be necessary beforehand — for example, is there anything I need to avoid?

- Are there any circumstances under which I should not have the test?

- Will it be done under sedation, local or general anaesthetic?

- Will any incision be needed to allow the scoping instrument to see the organ, and if so, how will this be performed?

- How painful will the test be?

- How long will the test take and when will the results be ready?

- What sort of after-care will be necessary?

The main types of scoping procedures include:

Arthroscopy: for the interior of a joint

Bronchoscopy: for the interior of the major air passages

Colonoscopy: for the interior lining of the large intestine (colon)

Colposcopy: for the cervix and vagina

Cystoscopy: for the interior lining of the bladder and urethra

Fetoscopy: for the developing foetus

Funduscopy: for the interior and back portions of the eye

Laparoscopy: for the outer surface of the abdominal organs (liver, intestines and spleen) and pelvic organs (uterus, fallopian tubes, and ovaries)

Laryngoscopy: for the base of the tongue, epiglottis, larynx and vocal cords

35

Mediastinoscopy: for the space behind the sternum and between the lungs which contains the heart and its major blood vessels, the windpipe, oesophagus and lymph nodes

Sigmoidoscopy: for the inside lining of the lower gastrointestinal tract (sigmoid colon, rectum and anus)

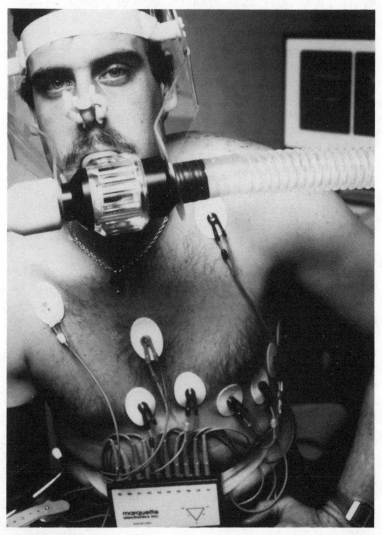

Figure 6. Equipment used in the computerized monitoring of cardiac fitness.

Upper gastrointestinal endoscopy: for the interior lining of the upper gastrointestinal tract

When scoping instruments are inserted into normal body openings the risks are minimal. However, there is a possibility of infection because of the difficulty in sterilizing the scope. If a previously detected pathology is present, there is the slight risk that the scope might perforate, rupture, or tear and cause bleeding of the organ being examined. When scopes are inserted through a surgical incision, there are the additional risks of surgery (ie problems with wound healing, wound herniation, and anaesthesia). The more appliances (brushes, biopsy cups, crushing clamps) that are attached to, or manipulated through a scope, the greater the risks. Since scoping procedures are invasive you should discuss the risks and benefits in detail with your doctor.

Because endoscopy involves the direct viewing of the organ or part of the viewing it is, when performed properly, 95% accurate. Most inaccuracies are due to insufficient training in the use of the endoscope.

PATHOLOGICAL TESTS

BIOPSY

Biopsy is the removal of a small piece of living tissue from an organ or part of the body for microscopic examination. It is an important tool in the diagnosis of cancer. A biopsy can be carried out as a separate diagnostic procedure, or during surgery or as part of an endoscopy.

There are three ways in which a biopsy can be performed:

Excision: This involves the complete removal of the lump, node or suspicious area and some of the surrounding tissue

Incision: When a small slice or wedge of the suspicious area is removed

Needle aspiration: where a long thin needle is inserted into the suspicious area and a small core of tissue removed

Once removed, the tissue is sent to a laboratory for analysis. If the biopsy takes place during surgery, the surgeon has a choice of actions:

Frozen section: the sample is rushed to the laboratory while the patient is still under anaesthetic. It is frozen, sliced and examined. Within 10 to 20 minutes the results are phoned through to the surgeon who then decides whether to remove further tissue or not, before bringing the patient round. If the results are positive, this can avoid a second operation. The sample deteriorates shortly after examination, so no second opinion is possible.

Permanent section: the sample is again sent to the laboratory but is prepared in such a way that the sample is permanently preserved. The patient is brought round, and then there is a discussion about whether any further surgery is necessary.

It is important that you discuss the two options with your doctor as there are clearly advantages and disadvantages to both. Nobody wants to go into the operating theatre believing the operation to be 'exploratory', and wake up minus an organ or limb.

Biopsies may be performed with no anaesthetic — such as those taken from the cervix under colpsocopy; whereas others will be performed under general anaesthetic. Pain and discomfort during and after, varies with what is being biopsied, and how. Ask your doctor what sort of biopsy you will be having, and why. Can such a major operation be avoided? And if not, what will it entail? As with other tests discuss with your doctor any preparation necessary, and anything that might affect the results.

General risk factors include the remote possibilities of haemorrhage and infection: much depends on the part of the body being biopsied. Many doctors feel that, when performing a biopsy on a suspected cancer, unless the biopsy is large enough to be outside the suspicious area, the irritation of the cutting or withdrawal of the biopsy needle may accelerate the spread of the cancer.

TAPS

Taps (or paracentesis) involve the process of drawing off excess fluid from a part of the body through a hollow needle or cannula (hollow tube containing a sharp pointed solid core which facilitates its insertion and is withdrawn when the cannula is in place). The fluid obtained is then sent for microscopic examination, chemical testing or culture. Analysis of the fluid is used to help determine whether infection, inflammation or cancer is present. A dry tap is one in which no fluid is obtained. A dry tap means either that there is no fluid in the target body cavity or that the fluid was missed.

Types of taps include:

Abdominal Tap: normally there is no fluid in the abdominal cavity, so its presence denotes certain conditions

Joint Tap: withdrawal of some of the lubricant surrounding the joint which increases under certain conditions causing painful swelling

Pleural Tap: under certain disorder fluid accumulates in the space between the lungs and the pleura

Spinal Tap: removal of cerebrospinal fluid which surrounds and cushions the brain and spinal cord — analysis of this fluid gives information about a variety of disorders affecting these organs (see Clinical Laboratory Tests)

All of these tests can be done on an out-patient basis, and are performed with, and sometimes without, local anaesthetic. The tests take between 5 to 20 minutes, depending on what is being tapped and are performed by a physician. The actual procedure varies so you should discuss with your doctor what will be done to you. There are slight risks of puncture of an organ by the needle, infection and bleeding. Certain patients may be at increased risk from a particular sort of tap, because of a condition they have, so you will be thoroughly tested before being passed for a tap. There may be some discomfort and pain during the tap, and there may be after effects — ask your doctor what to expect.

CYTOLOGY

Cytology tests detect and identify both normal and abnormal cells in areas that cannot be easily and directly examined. Cytology specimens include:

● **body excretions (urine, stools),**

● **secretions (sputum, gastric, eye, peritoneal, breast, prostatic, vaginal, and cerebrospinal fluid), and**

● **tissue scraping (uterus, vagina, mouth, nose, throat, bronchi, rectum, stomach, and cysts).**

They are mounted on slides and examined under a microscope. Cytology tests allow very early diagnosis of cancer as well as indicating hormone activity, specific infections and the effect of radiation. See Clinical Laboratory Tests for more details on collection of specimens.

SELF TESTS

There are now a wide range of home medical tests on the market: thermometers, pregnancy and fertility tests, blood pressure testing kits, vision and hearing testing kits, blood glucose monitoring systems, screening tests for colon cancer to name a few. Others, such as tests for monitoring blood cholesterol, urinary sodium and therapeutic drugs levels; and screening tests for sexually transmitted disease and breast cancer are under development.

In order for any of them to be effective in diagnosis, the instructions must be followed carefully. When used sensibly, such tests can help you evaluate symptoms and decide whether a visit to a doctor is necessary. However, you must remember that these tests are likely to be even less accurate than the tests carried out by professionals, so you may have an abnormal result even though you are quite healthy, or a home test may fail to detect some abnormality that is in fact present. You should always repeat the test, and if still unsure, seek medical advice. Some doctors suggest that if you are going to use home tests, try them on yourself and your family when you are healthy first; this will give you a base line reading and will also give you an opportunity to practise the technique. It may also be a good idea to discuss which tests are the best with your doctor.

CONCLUSION

Test results should only be used to confirm a diagnosis, not as the sole criteria in reaching a decision. Unfortunately the medical profession are becoming increasingly reliant on high technology, diagnostic techniques. No concomitant increase in diagnostic accuracy has been noted, but this has not stopped the exponential rise in the number of techniques being developed, marketed and used.

With so many diagnostic techniques available it is difficult for a patient to establish which are necessary, safe, or appropriate. Even if a technique has been shown to be reliable and safe, it may not be available in your area.

A radical rethink is needed, particularly in these economically difficult times. A detailed medical history and a physical examination can provide all the information a doctor requires. Doctors should ask themselves how many tests are really needed to confirm a diagnosis, and which test(s) would be the most appropriate to the patient under examination. Patients for their part, should ask why any technique has been recommended for them, and only agree to the test when they are happy with the information they have been given.

Chapter 3

THE ROLE OF PREVENTATIVE AND OCCUPATIONAL TESTS

PREVENTATIVE TESTS AND SCREENING

Preventative tests fall into two types: those which are performed on groups of people at risk, and those on people who are not at any known risk.

At present in the UK tests exist for the first category, namely those who are at risk by their work, through being pregnant or because they are children.

The value of tests performed in association with occupations is discussed below. In pregnancy the regular checks which are mentioned in the section on pregnancy have dramatically reduced the incidence of complications of pregnancy and early childhood. There has been a profound drop in infant mortality and in abnormal deliveries due to increasing antenatal care. The value of these tests is therefore undisputed.

Routine tests are carried out throughout childhood from the initial examination straight after birth to the reviews up to school age, and these are designed to be preventative in that they detect disease at an early stage before it becomes symptomatic or serious. They are also designed to check that normal growth and development is taking place so that any abnormalities can be rectified, and any adverse affects minimized. It is generally held that these regular checks and tests have led to a much healthier population with fewer problems which can be treated in early age.

PREVENTATIVE TESTS IN THE HEALTHY OR THOSE AT NO RISK

Whether regular check-ups and tests or screening for particular diseases are valuable in the normal adult population is a highly contentious and debatable issue. Many studies have been made, the majority of which have indicated that there is no value in regular checks. Some have shown that short examinations and some tests have some limited value, but one trial seemed to indicate that such regular checks can be positively harmful.

The value of screening is slightly less debatable, but it is important to recognize the difference between the regular check-up and screening.

The REGULAR CHECK-UP is the full examination of a healthy person combined with a number of standard medical tests. This is carried out at periodic intervals, sometimes annually, sometimes every three or five years.

SCREENING is when a specific test or examination on a group of the population or all the population (hopefully) is performed in order to try and identify a single disease or pre-symptomatic condition.

Let us consider first the value or otherwise of the medical check-up. It would seem that there are many and varied reasons for the performance of the regular check, only some of which may be significant. These are:

● Patients may be anxious that they have a particular condition, maybe because it tends to run in the family, or because they feel they are at particular risk.

● They are required to do so by their employer, for life insurance reasons etc.

● The patient just feels that it is a good thing to have a regular check-up for reassurance.

● The patient is convinced that preventative medicine is the ideal, and the check-up is an essential part of this programme.

Of the reasons given above, only the first is medical. If a patient is required to have a check by his employer for superannuation or insurance reasons, this may be more in the interests of the employer than the employee. It may ensure that the patient is fit to continue with his normal occupation, to the benefit of the company, and may also ensure that the company are not employing somebody who might become a financial liability by early retirement or premature illness.

Patients who simply feel that they should have one for reassurance are deluding themselves. A medical check can in no way of itself be preventative, and is not a guarantee that the patient will remain fit until the next check. These same reasons apply to patients who consider a check-up to be an essential part of a preventative medical programme.

The only type of patient who is justified in having an examination is the person who has a worry about a particular condition. However as this is regarding a specific condition rather than their general health, an examination along these lines comes into the area of screening, and the full examination and tests are therefore not required.

WHAT IS A 'FULL EXAMINATION'?

It is generally assumed, and accepted as standard practice by some insurance companies, that the full examination consists of a complete physical examination by a doctor, followed by routine tests. These include:

- Chest X-ray

- Electrocardiogram

- Full haematological blood analysis

- Full biochemical blood analysis

- Urinalysis (for protein, sugar, specific gravity and cells)

- Audiometry

- Spirometry (test of lung function)

- Visual test

45

- Test for blood in the stools (sometimes only if the patient is over 45)

- Weight and height checks

- Tonometry (check of the pressure within the eyeball)

It seems that this extensive range of investigations is considered by the patient to be essential, and if any one item were excluded then they would feel that they were not getting value. Unfortunately this tends to lead to a greater emphasis on the findings of the investigation, rather than the examination, and it has been previously mentioned that this is a potentially dangerous attitude.

Not all of the above tests are without risk, and many of the results can be established equally well by adequate physical examination. For example, it is now generally accepted that routine chest X-rays are more dangerous than is warranted by the number of positive findings which they show, and there are many conditions which affect the lungs which are not shown by X-ray, but which are detectable by the simple and harmless use of a stethoscope.

The electrocardiogram, whilst not dangerous, can provide a false sense of security. It tends to be assumed that if an ECG is normal, then the heart is in adequate condition and will remain so for the near future. Unfortunately this is not always the case, as shown by one study which revealed that half of the patients who died from coronary artery disease who had previously had a checkup in the last year, had not shown any sign of coronary heart disease at that check-up.

In addition it may be that some of the investigations give rise to unwarranted anxiety for the patient. One of the estimations taken for blood biochemical analysis is the serum uric acid. A raised uric acid level can be indicative of the tendency to develop gout. However at the time of examination, the patient may not have any symptoms of gout, but may develop some purely as a result of worry that they may have gout.

A number of investigations have been performed to try to estimate the value of regular medical check-ups and tests. One of the largest studies was undertaken in America in 1976 and was a controlled study in that a comparison was made between those who were checked on a regular basis, and those who were not. The patients were enrolled from all social classes and some were volunteers whereas others were encouraged to take part. A year after the initial examination, data was obtained from 84% of the sample, and any change in health was estimated. This was shown by a questionnaire, and by calculation of the number of days absence from work caused by illness and the number of visits to the doctor. It was found that there was no significant difference between the group that had been regularly examined and the unexamined group, except that interestingly the group which had been examined (possibly because they were therefore more aware of health factors) spent considerably more days in hospital.

In 1977, a study was made using the patients of a London Health Centre, who were all between 40 and 64 and who were identified and allocated to either a group which was tested and examined or to a group which was not. Both groups were of equal size. The tested group had the following examinations and tests performed:

- Health questionnaire

- Details of their occupation and occupational risks

- Height, weight and skin fold thickness tests

- Visual testing for near vision, distant vision and visual fields

- Audiometry

- Chest X-ray

- Lung function tests

- ECG

- Blood pressure

- Blood tests for haemoglobin, pack cell volume, blood urea, blood sugar, thyroid function and serum uric acid

- Examination of the stool for blood

- Examination of skin, mouth, teeth, joints, abdomen, legs, breast and pelvis.

After the initial examination, information was collected at six-monthly intervals on the basis of the number of consultations with their GP, hospital admission and periods of absence from work due to sickness, and deaths. A full investigation of the data was made some two years after the examination.

The results of this were interesting in that of the 3297 patients invited to attend, 73.4% did so. At the initial examination and test an average of 2.3 'diseases' per person was found. Furthermore just over half (53%) of this illness was previously unknown to the patient or the GP. Approximately 5% of the abnormalities discovered were considered to be clinically serious.

Some nine years later, the individuals were contacted to try and assess the data by comparing it with their health since. It was found that of the two groups there was no significant difference in either the prevalence of symptoms or disability, of GP consultation rates, or rates for hospital admission. Indeed, the only significant finding of the study was that there was a consistently higher mortality rate in those who had initially refused to enter the trial.

It would seem from this study that simple advice regarding social habits (e.g. diet, smoking and drinking) may well have greater effect on health than regular medical checks. Obviously the patient himself knows whether he is overweight, drinking excessively or smoking too much, and only needs the support and advice of a medical expert, but not complicated and expensive tests. One study performed in 1977 did suggest that there might indeed be a positively harmful effect from regular medical checks. Out of a group of steel workers, 208 were found to have high blood pressure. Seventy of these had previously known that they were hypertensive. In the following year, there was 80% increase in days off sick in the patients who had been told that they had blood pressure problems. In addition to this there was the anxiety and possible hazards, previously mentioned, by the regular examination and unwarranted medical test.

Clearly for the tests to be valid, they must fulfil certain criteria.

● They must satisfy the patient's personal needs.

● They must not be repetitious (it is for example, useless to test for colour blindness more than once).

● They must be thorough in that no test which could be of value should be omitted.

SCREENING

Screening, on the other hand, provided certain factors are borne in mind, may well be beneficial. The condition which one is trying to demonstrate must:

- have a definite pre-clinical or pre-symptomatic stage.

- must be amenable to treatment at the stage at which it is detected.

In addition, the screening programme must:

- be significant in terms of reduced illness or reduced death rates.

- be significant in improvement of the health of the population as a whole.

One factor that must be borne in mind when attempting to set up a screening programme is the value or otherwise of the test. There are a number of tests which would appear to show an abnormality, when in fact none is present. This is known as a false positive test, and the rate of false positives varies according to the test. Visual testing can be over 30% false positive, spirometry 29% false positive, audiometry 23% false positive, and even blood pressure tests can be 6.2% false positive. Interestingly the test with the lowest false positives appears to be the ECG with only 0.1%.

In addition one has to bear in mind that some tests will appear negative when the disease or condition is actually present. False negative tests have been less examined than false positive tests, but as previously mentioned, over half the people dying of cancer and heart disease within a year of the test had not shown any sign of their condition at the examination.

In addition to the factors listed above, the disease which one is attempting to discover must clearly be prevalent to make the testing economically viable. In the 1950s, regular mass screening by chest X-ray was undertaken in order to discover early tuberculosis. This was successful not only in that it resulted in earlier treatment for the patient, but it also reduced the incidence in the general population by spread of the infection. However in the 1980s tuberculosis is so uncommon that mass screening would be inappropriate in view of its expense.

At the moment the only screening tests performed with central government support are cervical and breast screening. The former appears to have resulted in a reduction in cervical cancer; however there are inadequacies in the system when it comes to following up at risk patients. However, the incidence of cervical cancer has been steadily decreasing since 1946, quite irrespective of the introduction of cervical smear screening. It remains to be seen how valuable the breast screening programme will be.

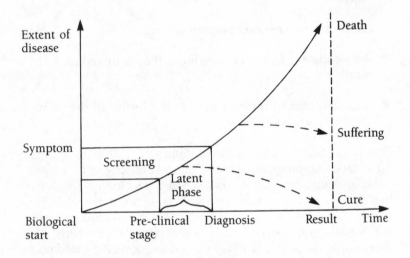

Figure 7. The values of early screening.

Figure 7 indicates the possible value of early screening. The stage between the time when early diagnosis is possible and the diagnosis being made (known as the latent phase, when it is detectable by laboratory methods, but before symptoms actually occur) varies from disease to disease. After the symptoms have developed, clearly the patient would go and see the doctor, and is then out of range for a screening service. Within the latent phase, screening may be possible and treatment effect the cure (as shown by the dotted line).

Unfortunately, the latent phase varies from disease to disease, and may be only a matter of weeks in some conditions or many years in others. Obviously for a screening programme to be effective and useful, the condition being examined must have a long latent phase.

One example of the potentially useful screening system is the regular check-up (known as tonometry) for glaucoma or increased blood pressure within the eye. If the pressure builds up within the eye, damage to the retina can occur, resulting in tunnel vision, where the visual field is reduced to a small area around the point at which the eye is fixed. This develops insidiously over a number of years, and when noticed by the patient, recovery may be impossible. Tonometry, on the other hand, is easy, cheap (with the advent of new instruments), quick and totally without risk.

It is often suggested that blood pressure may also be worth while screening for in that it develops without symptoms, and often produces disease (for example, strokes or arteriosclerosis). Once again the test is without risk, quick and cheap.

To sum up, the evidence at the moment for regular medical check-ups on the normal healthy adult is inconclusive, but tends to show that there is no long-term benefit other than reassurance to the patient (which may be unwarranted). Screening is valuable for specific conditions, but check-ups as already initiated in this country for children, pregnant women and people in particular occupations continues to be of value.

OCCUPATIONAL HEALTH AND HEALTH TESTS

In the UK medical examinations and tests for workers figure prominently in the occupational health services: periodic medical examinations are seen to offer some preventative health advantage. It will now be clear, in view of the remarks made above, that unless workers are exposed to particular risks, the benefits from such regular medical examinations are of minimal use, as the value of information obtained from routine medical examination and tests is generally over estimated.

In addition, little attempt is made to differentiate between screening and case finding. Screening aims to divide the population into two groups, those with a higher and those with a lower probability of being affected by certain medical conditions. Case finding on the other hand is the detection of a particular disease common in a particular working group by means of various tests. It has recently been suggested that there are only a few adult conditions that are worth the trouble of regular surveillance in occupational examinations. These include:

- Infectious diseases such as German measles, cholera, tuberculosis, hepatitis etc.

- Visual defects, including primary glaucoma

- Diabetes

- Hypothyroidism (under-active thyroid gland)

- Raised blood pressure

- Chronic bronchitis

- Cancer of the breast, cervix, colon and rectum, bladder and skin

- Dental caries

Medical examinations might also be useful in attempts to alter an individual's lifestyle or habits (for example, reduction of smoking and alcohol consumption) but it seems that this has a poor response rate.

Regular medical examinations, however, can form part of a useful occupational health practice if they are only undertaken for specific reasons and with specific objectives in mind. It should also be remembered that specific consequent actions dependent on the results must be expected.

Some medical examinations may be statutory, for example, for workers in occupations exposed to radiation. Most examinations are voluntary, however, and are either pre-work or periodic, usually after a period of sickness, within a specific occupations group, or before retirement.

PRE-WORK EXAMINATIONS AND TESTS

These can be useful if they are required or useful for the following reasons:

- to assess whether an individual is fit to do the job specified (for example, heavy goods vehicle drivers).

- to assess overall fitness for any occupation.

- to detect existing ill health which may be treated to allow the applicant to do a specific job, or the job may be adjusted to the individual's health requirements.

- for the purpose of pension fund or insurance.

- to find suitable work for disabled people.

The most efficient way of conducting pre-work or pre-employment examinations, is to divide them into four stages.

Stage one: A health questionnaire is filled in by the prospective employee.

Stage two: A nurse performs some additional tests such as blood pressure, urine tests, simple blood tests and checks in vision and hearing.

Stage three: A doctor makes an examination.

Stage four: Further, more specialized, investigations are conducted.

Most employees will only need to pass through stages one and two, and this is sufficient in practice for 90% of prospective employees. The nurse might only pass on any who show an abnormality in the basic tests, those who give concern from their health questionnaire or those in specific occupations. These might include:

- those concerned with public safety, for example, drivers of public service vehicles

- employees in physically exceptionally strenuous jobs, for example, divers

- employees who are to be exposed to potentially toxic or physiologically active agents.

Generally, this series of examinations and tests will suffice to either adapt the job to suit the applicant, or to treat the applicant to suit the job. Unfortunately, confused and rather varying opinion can rest on these tests, particularly where superannuation and insurance schemes are involved. There is one large employer in Britain who will not employ any insulin dependent diabetic, as from experience, they have found that such persons have a poorer absence record, and tend to retire early. On the other hand, when it was pointed out to the same employer that the same reasons could be applied for not employing any smokers, this was dismissed.

OCCUPATIONAL HISTORY

The first pre-requisite for any medical examination or test concerned with future employment must be the previous occupational history. All too often when taking a medical history from a patient, this aspect is ignored, and vague descriptions of occupations such as 'retired' or 'sedentary' are included. Greater details regarding a patient's previous occupation may well give a clue to the cause of an existing complaint.

Any account of occupational history should include information on the following:

- how long the patient has been at that particular job

- the hours of work

- a description of the work done

- whether there was any exposure to dust, fumes, gases, excessive temperatures, noise, radiation, infectious agents. Whether the job involved undue stress and other psychological factors.

There should be a note of any hobbies which account for a number of hours of the patient's time, as these may be significant (for example, bird fanciers' lung in bird breeders).

POST SICKNESS ABSENCE EXAMINATIONS AND TESTS

Of all employment medical examinations, this is probably the most valuable, in that it allows the doctor to examine the employee in the light of the job in which he is performing, and to assess this, bearing in mind the illness which he has recently suffered. Such examinations can provide clues to the cause of disease in industry and consequent changes of practices can be to the benefit of all the employees.

There is considerable variation amongst companies regarding the exact requirements for a personal examination and test after illness, but it is generally speaking good practice if examination takes place under the following circumstances:

- any absence for sickness longer than four weeks

- any absence after an accident at work

- any absence due to cancer, heart disease, neurological disease, infectious disease (in food handlers) and psychiatric disorders.

PERIODIC MEDICAL EXAMINATIONS AND TESTS FOR SPECIFIC VULNERABLE GROUPS

Such tests should not take the place of post sickness examinations, but may in some cases be useful, and are sometimes mandatory.

DRIVERS

Drivers of public service vehicles and heavy goods vehicles are required by law to be examined on their appointment and at specific periods thereafter. The exact timing of these examinations and tests varies from company to company, but in some it is every year, and others every four or five years. Clearly their effectiveness depends upon the co-operation of the employee being examined, and specifically agreed procedures within the company should be adhered to, such that any adverse medical reports do not adversely affect the employee's income.

SPECIFIC AGE GROUPS

The very young and very old may require specific medical review at times, although the statutory examination of young persons has now been abolished. Such examinations might occasionally have a place in some occupations in view of the psychological stresses of adjustment between school and work. For much the same reasons, pre-retirement medical examinations and tests may be helpful in adjustment between working life and retirement.

WOMEN

It is often considered that women are more vulnerable than men, and hence they are subject to periodic examinations and tests. There is little to support this practice, as they are usually more resilient than men, and certainly have longer lifespan. The only working factor which might be detrimental to them, is the contact with any toxic agents which might damage a child they were carrying. Workers in such occupations may therefore need periodic screening throughout their reproductive lives.

FOOD HANDLERS

Clearly those whose occupations involve the handling of food are not risks to themselves but to the consumers of their products. An applicant for a food handling job might be disqualified on the grounds of:

● inflammation of the ear or infection of the eye

● persistent skin conditions which are subject to infection (e.g. impetigo)

● persistent respiratory disease (e.g. tuberculosis)

● a history of typhoid or paratyphoid disease

- an intestinal disease in which absence of pathological bacteria has not been excluded

Clearly it is also essential to have a medical review and tests if necessary before such workers return to work after an absence due to sickness.

EXECUTIVES

It has recently become almost accepted practice within many companies for the top executives to have regular annual screening medicals. Apart from providing some unwarranted peace of mind to the applicant, there is little justification for the many examinations which are performed. These screening methods have been the subject of many controlled trials, which show that the numerous tests to which the executive is subjected have little value in terms of prognosis. For any test to be of value the following criteria are important:

- The condition for which the test is made should be an important health problem.

- The cost should be economical.

- The condition should have a recognizable pre-symptomatic stage.

- Facilities for treatment and aids for accepted treatment should be available.

- The test should be without risk or have a risk level which is acceptable to the patient.

It is therefore clear that it is impossible to lay down specific guidelines for the monitoring of occupational disease or screening programmes. In many companies simple screening carried out by a nurse can be effective in the majority of cases, reducing the time necessary for a doctor. Only a minimum of those who have to see the doctor should require any extensive tests, and these should almost always be related to the occupation and not standardized.

ROLE OF BIOLOGICAL MONITORING

Biological monitoring is the regular measuring of toxic substances in a patient's body to which he or she is exposed through his or her occupation. Clearly this is only going to be of use where the monitoring levels are standardized and accepted (a recent test showed that estimation of serum lead levels on the same sample ranged in laboratories between 100 micrograms per litre and 1200 micrograms per litre) and if the substance which is toxic causes a condition which can be prevented by treatment in the early stage. Once again, as with all medical tests, it is very important that a test is used for the right reasons, and any possible errors known about.

The following points need to be borne in mind when considering biological monitoring:

- Biological monitoring is not a substitute for environmental monitoring. Environmental monitoring assesses the risk, and biological monitoring the result of a risk that has not been adequately controlled.

- The substance which is to be examined must be present in some tissue or blood fluid.

- Valid and accurate methods for analysis must be available.

- The measurements must be correct.

- The acceptable levels of the suspect agent must be standardized in terms of the maximum permissible.

Because of factors in the patient's home environment as well as the working environment, the results for a group of workers may have more significance than for individuals.

Whether or not to test the substance itself must also be considered, as must whether or not to examine that part of the body exposed to the substance (for example, if a person has been exposed to radiation, effect on the blood cells).

It is obviously necessary to have a maximum level of each substance which is permissible, and the World Health Organization has laid out the following recommended values:

Substance	Recommended Value	Comments
Lead (in blood)	400 mcg per 100mls 300 mcg per 100mls	in males in females of reproductive age
Cadmium (in urine)	10 mcg per 100gms of creatinine excreted	
Cadmium (in blood)	10 mcg per 100mls	
Mercury (in urine)	50 mcg per 100 mls	estimated as a group
Arsenic (in urine)	100 mcg per 100mls	
Trichloroacetic acid (in urine)	50mgs per 100gms of creatinine	a group average at the end of the working day
Carboxy-haemoglobin	2.5%-3%	this applies to the general population as well as to workers who are exposed to carbon monoxide.

There may also be a place for examining certain target organs which are known to be damaged in particular occupations. An obvious example of this are regular chest X-rays to detect the existence of asbestosis in patients exposed to asbestos through their work. Some further examples of organs affected in similar ways include the following:

● The lungs — workers whose occupation exposes them to dusts such as flour, fungi, wood dust, formalin, dyes, adhesive fumes, coal, silica, feathers (in these patients, the problem may be an allergy or a direct toxic effect from the substance on the lung).

- The nervous system — mercury compounds, lead and compounds, arsenic, antimony, pesticides.

- The bladder and kidney — chloroform, carbon tetrachloride, phenol, turpentine, insecticides, cadmium.

- The heart and blood vessels — trichoroethylene, carbon tetrachloride, halothane, fluorocarbons, vinyl, carbon monoxide.

- The skin — epoxy resins, rubber, nickel, mercury, plants (primula, daffodil, chrysanthemum), hardwoods, pharmaceuticals.

- The liver — carbon tetrachloride, insecticides, alcohols, phenol

- The endocrine system — anaesthetic gasses, vinyl, lead, hormones.

Regular occupational health checks, if correctly performed as discussed above, can be helpful in that they ensure the continuing health of the employee to both his benefit and to the benefit of the company.

Chapter 4

MAJOR DISEASES, INFECTIONS AND CONDITIONS

DEGENERATIVE DISEASES

CYSTIC FIBROSIS

Cystic fibrosis is a hereditary disease that affects the exocrine glands (including the sweat and mucus producing glands); the lungs; intestines; bile duct and pancreas. In 1985 the cystic fibrosis gene was located. As a result, prenatal screening is now available to high risk couples as early as the first trimester. The screening technique used is chorionic villi sampling (see Chapter 5). The DNA in the sample is analysed. There is a 5% risk of a false negative result using this technique. Alternatively cystic fibrosis can be detected in the foetus using amniocentesis (see Chapter 5) to measure three isoenzymes of alkaline phosphatase.

In order to diagnose cystic fibrosis after birth, there are a number of tests available:

SWEAT TESTS

This is the most commonly performed test (see Chapter 2 for details), taking between 40 and 60 minutes, and with the advantage of not being painful, if performed properly. A child with cystic fibrosis will have abnormally high levels of sodium and chloride in his or her sweat.

Mothers can perform a crude sweat test by kissing or licking their baby's skin, and then their own. If the baby's skin tastes highly salty it suggests that the baby may have cystic fibrosis. This should not, however, be taken as a definitive diagnosis and professional advice should be sought.

Sweat measurements are reasonably significant as a confirmation of cystic fibrosis. Inaccuracies are usually due to the carelessness of the tester. There are some doctors who maintain that the sweat test is of no real value until a baby is more than six weeks old.

BLOOD TESTS

Immunoreactive Trypsin Assay: This test is used to detect the presence of trypsin, a digestive enzyme produced by the pancreas. When an individual has cystic fibrosis, mucus blocks the pancreatic ducts and trypsin retreats into the blood and can be detected there. This test can be performed on babies who are only a few weeks old. See Chapter 2 for more details.

Immunological Reactive Trypsinogen (IRT) test: This is a new test based on pancreatic secretions and can help detect cystic fibrosis within the first week of life. If the result is positive, the test is repeated after a month.

RADIOGRAPHY

A chest X-ray can highlight some of the symptoms of cystic fibrosis.

STOOLS MICROSCOPY

A stools specimen is analysed for the fat content as one method of confirmation of cystic fibrosis.

ANALYSIS OF SPUTUM

As with stools, the analysis of sputum can provide confirmation of the diagnosis of cystic fibrosis. See Chapter 2 for more details.

PANCREATIC FUNCTION TESTS

These are used in the diagnosis of older patients, as the sweat test becomes less reliable with the increasing age of the individual.

PARKINSON'S DISEASE

A person with Parkinson's disease is suffering from disturbances of brain function due to the chemical imbalance in certain nerve cells near the base of the brain. This produces the symptoms which characterize the disorder.

- involuntary shaking movements of the limbs (tremor)

- stiffness of the muscles (rigidity), and

- a slowness and poverty of spontaneous movements (bradykinesia).

These can be abated if the chemical imbalance is redressed with drugs. Its onset begins in middle or old age and in many cases no cause can be found. Certain drugs are known to induce Parkinsonism, and more rarely its occurrence has been attributed to the late effects of encephalitis or coal-gas poisoning or to Wilson's disease.

There is no specific laboratory test which becomes positive in the presence of Parkinson's disease. Blood tests, X-rays, and brain scans (see Chapter 2) may be performed — but these are essentially to exclude other causes rather than to make a positive diagnosis. Diagnosis is made solely by consideration of an individual's symptoms and incapacities through interview and physical examination. The onset of Parkinsonism is slow, the initial symptoms appearing almost imperceptibly. They are often vague and non-specific — such as inexplicable tiredness, mildly aching muscles and cramps. Therefore, regular evaluation of a patient plays an important part in the diagnosis and management of patients with Parkinson's disease.

MUSCULAR DYSTROPHY

Muscular dystrophy refers to a group of muscle diseases in which there is a recognizable pattern of inheritance. They are characterized by weakness and wasting of selected muscles: the affected muscle fibres degenerate and are replaced by fatty tissue. The muscular dystrophies are classified according to the:

- patient's age at onset

- distribution of the weakness

- progression of the disease, and

- mode of inheritance.

Diagnosis of muscular dystrophy utilizes the following tests:

CREATINE PHOSPHOKINASE (CPK)

This is a blood test (see Chapter 2) in which the levels of CPK in the blood serum are measured. CPK is an enzyme that is found mainly in skeletal muscle, heart muscle, and the brain. When muscle is damaged, CPK leaks into the bloodstream and can be detected there. There are at least three forms of CPK, called iso-enzymes. They are labelled according to where they are primarily found: heart muscle, and brain:

- CPK-1 is the brain isoenzyme

- CPK-2 (CPK-MB) is the heart isoenzyme

- CPK-3 is the muscle isoenzyme

Measuring CPK levels can be used to indicate muscular dystrophy and to follow the progress of the illness. Total CPK increases are associated with muscular dystrophy, but also with

- hypothyroidism

- alcoholism

- crush injury of the muscles

- asthma and other lung conditions that make breathing difficult

- heart attack (coronary).

Because so many conditions are indicated by an increase in total CPK, this test is not very specific — and is considered about 70% accurate.

ELECTROMYOGRAPHY (EMG)

EMG measures the electrical activity in muscles, and can be used to investigate the cause of weakness or paralysis.

NERVE CONDUCTION STUDIES

Nerve conduction studies measure the ability of specific nerves to transmit electrical impulses. As with EMG, nerve conduction studies can be used to investigate the cause of weakness or paralysis.

MUSCLE BIOPSY

Muscle biopsy can be used to confirm the diagnosis of muscular dystrophy. However such a biopsy is rarely required when symptoms and signs are present. It is only really used to diagnose very early or atypical cases.

SCREENING

Through the use of chromosome analysis of the blood and Chorionic Villi sampling (see Chapter 5) it is possible to identify carriers of Duchenne muscular dystrophy (most common form of this disorder) by the third month of pregnancy. This is said to be more accurate than total CPK measurement.

MULTIPLE SCLEROSIS

Multiple sclerosis (MS) is a chronic disease of the nervous system that affects young and middle aged adults. Its cause is unknown, but there is evidence that points to the sufferer's abnormal response to viral infection. There also appears to be a genetic element that increases an individual's susceptibility to MS, but which does not operate through direct inheritance.

The myelin sheaths (insulating layer of protein and phospholipid) surrounding nerves in the brain and spinal cord are damaged as a result of MS. This affects the function of these nerves. MS is characterized by recurrent relapses followed by remission. The disease affects different parts of the brain and spinal cord which in turn results in typically scattered symptoms — in location and time. These include:

● unsteady gait

● shaky movements of the limbs (ataxia)

● rapid involuntary movements of the eyes (nystagmus)

● defects in speech pronunciation (dysarthria)

● spastic weakness

● retrobulbar neuritis (inflammation of the optic nerve)

Diagnosis of MS is notoriously difficult — depending as it does on a pattern of symptoms and signs occurring over a period of time — often years. Because in the early stages of MS many of the symptoms clear up after a short period (remission) they may be forgotten or ignored. The symptoms are also rather general — such as numbness or tingling — and if they occur without any obvious impairment to reflexes, a GP may dismiss the individual's fears as 'hysterical' — particularly if the person is a woman.

There are a handful of other conditions that have similar symptoms to MS, but these are mostly quite rare. Syphilis of the nervous system is one which can easily be eliminated through a simple blood test. The most common source of error is to confuse severe MS with a benign tumour compressing the spinal cord. This sort of tumour can be removed and a complete recovery effected. Because of this it is often necessary to carry out X-rays to ensure that no such mistake has been made.

Spinal cord damage can also be caused by a deficiency of vitamin B12 — usually resulting from pernicious anaemia. Again this can be diagnosed by a blood test, and the deficiency rectified.

There is no specific test for MS. For a diagnosis doctors have mainly had to rely on interview and physical examination. The following tests are currently used to confirm the diagnosis, but none are sufficiently accurate or specific to provide a diagnosis in isolation:

ANALYSIS OF THE CEREBRO-SPINAL FLUID (CSF)

A sample of CSF is collected by a lumbar puncture (see Chapter 2 for details). This technique is not without risks, and some doctors argue that it can precipitate relapse in MS. The following changes in the CSF are indicative of MS:

- Slightly higher level of white blood cells and protein are found in about 50% of MS sufferers. These changes are inconstant and are also found in many other forms of organic nervous disease.

- The proportion of protein present in the form of globulin increases. However, even this change is only found in about 70% of cases, and is also present in other diseases. Some more refined techniques of examination of the globulin in the CSF have shown abnormalities in more than 90% of patients with MS. But again, similar changes are found in some patients with other diseases.

EVOKED POTENTIALS

It is now possible to record from the surface of the skin the minute electrical potentials induced or evoked by a specific stimulus. This technique is similar to that described under nerve conduction studies (muscular dystrophy). Any damage to the myelin sheath of the nerves under investigation will result in a delay in nerve conduction. For example, it was shown that even after the eye affected by retrobulbar neuritis had recovered, there was still a delay in conduction — thus supplying doctors with a method of detecting the effects of MS in the absence of relevant symptoms.

A sufficiently high number of abnormal EP readings from different nerves have been found in known MS sufferers, to warrant the use of the technique on patients in whom the diagnosis is in doubt. However, at best a positive result has been obtained in only two thirds of MS sufferers.

CT SCAN

CT scans of the brain are sometimes performed as they can show areas of the brain that have been damaged by MS. Their role is still being defined, but it is clear that in the future CT scans may become more useful in diagnosis and indeed the monitoring of MS.

HOT BATH TEST

This technique can be used to determine the cause of suspicious neurological manifestations since most MS sufferers experience an increase in the severity of their symptoms and muscle problems when their body temperature rises. A hot bath is used to deliberately raise your body temperature. You first lie in a bath with the water temperature at 100°F or 38°C. Then the temperature is raised a degree at a time while the arms, legs and especially the eyes are closely observed. Within 15 minutes, the temperature reaches 110°F or 43°C at which point it is cooled to starting temperature. Blood pressure and pulse measurements are also recorded. When the water temperature is raised more than one degree, MS sufferers experience various signs and symptoms of the disease — either for the first time or, if they had been present before, to a much worse degree.

However it has been known for the symptoms to persist for more than 24 hours after the test, and there have been reports of permanent or prolonged neurological complications in some patients after undergoing the hot bath test. About 60% of patients with MS will experience MS symptoms when hot-bathed compared with only 1% of those not suffering from MS. This test is rarely used as a routine diagnostic measure.

FIELD TESTS

There are a series of diagnostic tests on samples of blood (named after their author) that have been claimed to be absolutely specific for MS. Further, they are claimed as a reliable screening technique — detecting those susceptible to MS from early childhood. The tests are based on the hypothesis that in MS, cell membranes in all tissues are abnormal as a result of a congenital disorder of fatty acid metabolism. This is hotly contested. In studies so far carried out no consistent results were achieved. The most promising test is the E-UFA test (erythrocyte-unsaturated fatty acid). Red blood cells are tested by electrophoresis to note changes in the motility. However, no real agreement has been reached on a consistently repeatable methodology; until it is reached it is unlikely that this test will be commonly used or even available in hospitals in this country.

CONCLUSION

Degenerative diseases are distressing and debilitating, not only to the sufferer, but also their friends and relatives. While the outlook is still rather bleak, advances are being made in early diagnosis and even in genetic counselling for 'at risk' parents contemplating a family. Earlier diagnosis can help in providing better, more effective treatment; and genetic counselling can at least give parents information on their chances of producing an unaffected child. It is also to be hoped that the treatments available will improve with greater understanding of the disease processes, achieved through research.

URINARY TRACT INFECTIONS AND DISORDERS

The urinary tract is a broad term used to describe the organs, ducts and channels that are involved in the passing of urine from the kidneys out of the body. This includes the ureters, the bladder and the urethra. Adjacent organs such as the prostate and epididymis are usually included in the definition.

URINARY TRACT INFECTIONS

Infections of the urinary tract are caused by variety of infectious agents including bacteria and viruses. They can gain access to the urinary tract via the bloodstream, but more commonly they enter from outside up the urethra into the bladder.

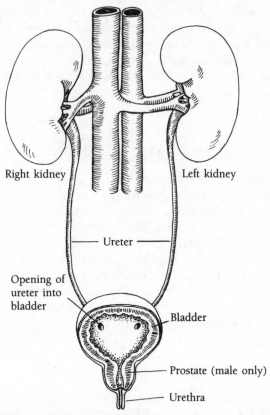

Figure 8. Diagram showing the organs of the urinary tract.

Urine is a very good medium for bacteria to multiply in, particularly given the warm temperature inside our bodies which encourages their growth. The increase in bacteria is not always accompanied by symptoms, but the most common ones that are likely to propel you to your doctor include:

● pain around the bladder area

● severe burning hot pain during and just after passing urine

● frequent urination, followed by the immediate desire to urinate again

● blood in the urine, and

● **fever, with or without a shivering attack.**

Urinary tract infections cannot be definitively diagnosed clinically (through interview and examination) so confirmation is required from laboratory tests.

The first, and most important investigation of known or suspected urinary tract infection is to *culture the urine*. Urine may also be examined microscopically. So, whether you are at your GP's surgery, a clinic or hospital you will be asked to provide a sample of urine. You will be given a sterile container and asked to collect a *midstream specimen* of urine (MSU). This sample is representative of the true microbiological situation in the bladder, because the discarded first volume of urine will have washed away any micro-organisms in the urinary tract that might have contaminated the specimen. If for any reason, investigation of the germs in the urethra is required, the first volume of urine may be collected as a specimen.

Collecting a MSU can be impossible for individuals who have poor control of bladder emptying: babies, young children, elderly women, and patients with neropathic bladders or ileal bladders, in which case, there are two other methods of urine collection:

SUPRAPUBIC ASPIRATION

You are asked to lie on a couch, and a small section of your lower abdomen is cleansed with antiseptic. A needle is then inserted into the bladder through the abdominal wall, and urine is collected through the needle. This test is performed by a physician and, surprisingly, is almost painless.

CATHETERIZATION

A thin sterilised, but lubricated tube (catheter) is passed into the bladder through the urethra, while you are lying on a couch. A sample from the bladder can then be taken directly. There is a risk of infection using this method if the catheter is not properly sterilised and inserted.

If a sample of urine from the kidney is required, a catheter is inserted and the bladder is then washed with sterile irrigating fluid to remove any micro-organisms that might contaminate the urine as it arrives from the kidney. A drug may also be passed into the bladder to kill any micro-organisms. Then timed samples of urine are collected for analysis.

It is important that the sample is set up for culture as soon as possible — preferably within half an hour of collection. Organisms from the urethral opening may grow in urine if it is left standing at room temperature, and other organisms which are genuine infecting agents may die off. Delay in getting specimens to the laboratory is a major reason for inaccurate diagnoses and subsequently ineffective treatment. If doctors are unable to get specimens straight to the laboratory, they will usually refrigerate them until they can be processed. You should check with your doctor where and when the results will be available, as this varies. They should come through very quickly in order that you can be put onto the correct treatment if no interim medication has been given, or to change your medication if it is inappropriate. However, the onus will be on you to find out your results — you will not usually be notified.

Having identified the organism, and established the right treatment, a doctor then has to decide whether further investigation is necessary.

URINARY TRACT DISORDERS

The object of further investigation is to determine whether, in addition to the infection, you have some underlying abnormality of the kidneys or the urinary tract. A doctor will usually only recommend further investigation if you have a history of recurrent urinary infections.

Methods of further investigation (see Chapter 2 for details of each technique) include:

BLOOD TESTS

Used to estimate the level of various substances concerned directly with renal function (urea, creatine, phosphate, uric acid) and other substances which relate to the kidney's regulatory capacity (such as the electrolytes sodium and potassium). Do not be alarmed at the amount of blood that is taken for analysis — you do have 12 pints!

24 HOUR URINE COLLECTION

This can be a nuisance to collect, as you have to carry the collection bottle around with you everywhere. Do follow the doctor's instructions, and tell him/her if you miss a collection — as (s)he can then take this into consideration when analysing the specimen. 24 hour urine samples are usually required for estimation of protein loss, creatine clearance, calcium and or sodium excretion — all important factors in kidney functioning.

X-RAYS

of the kidney (IVP): The doctor will want to ensure that your bowels are empty of gas because it may obscure the pictures. If your kidney function is normal, or nearly normal, you will be asked to restrict your fluid intake prior to the X-ray to ensure concentrated urine. Contrast material will be injected into your arm — this can be unpleasant if large doses are used. Pictures are then taken shortly after the injection, up to two hours later, and one after the bladder has been emptied.

of the bladder (micturating cystogram): this is a rather trying and embarrassing test for the patient, but one which provides much valuable information for doctor. A sterile catheter is passed into the bladder, and radio-opaque contrast material passed in. The catheter is then removed and you are asked to urinate, whilst still or cine pictures of the bladder and urethra are taken. This is not easy to do with an audience! Pressure measurements may be taken at the same time from the bladder and rectum — using very fine probes.

of the blood vessels to the kidney (renal angiogram): You will have to lie quietly during this test, but you will be given premedication which will make you sleepy or even send you to sleep during the procedure. Under local anaesthetic, fine catheters are passed into the large blood vessels in the groin, and manipulated up to the kidney inside the vessel. Radio-opaque contrast material is then injected into the kidney (and blood samples taken if needed from the kidney). After the test, pressure is maintained on the blood vessels and you will have to remain in bed to allow the tiny punctures in the blood vessels to heal. This means you will probably spend a night in hospital.

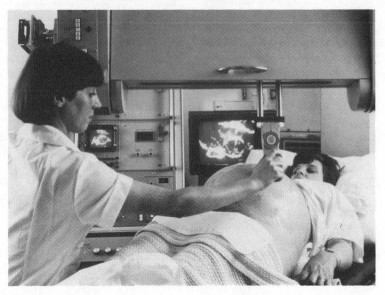

Figure 9. A pregnant woman is examined by ultrasound.

CT SCANS

Scans, particularly those using radioisotopes, are being used more and more in preference to standard X-rays in order to investigate kidney disorders. The radioisotope used is either one which will 'home in' on the kidney, or one that passes through the kidney.

ULTRASOUND

This technique can be used to produce a picture of what is going on inside the kidney, the entrance to the ureters, and the bladder surface.

Ultrasound can also be used to evaluate obstructions in the upper tracts and detecting patterns of flow of blood and urine.

KIDNEY BIOPSY

This has been an important technique for patients with glomerular disease. The procedure requires you to spend at least two nights in hospital in order for you to rest while the puncture to the kidney heals.

CONCLUSION

Urinary tract infection is a common condition, especially in women — because of the shorter urethra, but rarely indicates a more serious disorder.

TOXICOLOGY

Toxicology is the study of potentially poisonous materials and their effects upon living organisms. This section considers the tests related to three aspects of toxicology:

DRUG ABUSE

A drug is abused when it is taken intentionally by an individual for a desired non-medical effect, or when taken in overdose. The drugs most commonly abused include the amphetamines, alcohol, barbiturates, narcotic analgesics, hallucinogens, and benzodiazepines.

In the past it has been difficult to detect the presence of any of these drugs, but there are now quick, simple tests for detecting their presence in urine (see Chapter 2). These tests are primarily used for screening, and as such have proved extremely effective. They can be performed by anyone, at any location, but if there are any legal implications attached to the testing (possible prosecution for example), urine or blood samples are sent to laboratories for more complex biochemical blood or urine analysis to ensure greater accuracy. The accuracy of these tests varies. If properly performed they are more than 90% accurate, but the overall accuracy — when screening large population groups such as the military, is only about 33%. False positives have been reported, and false negatives are common — even when testing for marihuana, which should still be detected after three weeks.

Providing a urine sample for either sort of analysis presents no medical risk to the patient — except that of providing self-incriminating evidence.

THERAPEUTIC DRUG MONITORING

Drugs are potent, whether prescribed or abused; and there is only a fine line between safety and toxicity. Added to this, individuals vary in their response to drugs. There are therefore many clinical situations in which drug monitoring is, or should be, employed. These include:

- determining the optimum dose of a therapeutic drug in order to avoid adverse effects

- when there is doubt that a patient is taking the prescribed drug

- in the diagnosis of pathological conditions resulting from accidental or intentional exposure to toxic substances

- helping in the clinical management of patients threatened by the use or abuse of drugs, or whose response to a given drug therapy is inappropriate

In most instances a blood sample is taken from a vein (see Chapter 2) and the serum tested. Substances are usually considered toxic when their serum concentrations become great enough to produce deleterious effects. Samples of urine, body tissues, stomach contents and hair or nail shavings can also be tested.

Drugs are generally administered in a set dose, at regular intervals, and over an extended period of time. This allows the serum drug concentration to rise gradually to therapeutic concentrations. The serum concentration range is known as the 'steady-state condition'. There is a constant fluctuation within this, between a high (peak) and low (trough) value for drug concentration.

With such fluctuations, it is important that blood or urine samples are taken at the right time. In order to establish that a patient is indeed getting a therapeutic dose of the drug, a blood sample should be taken shortly before the next dose is due. If toxicity is suspected sampling should occur shortly after the dose was taken, when there is a maximum drug concentration in the serum (peak). It is essential that the doctor is as consistent as possible with the sampling time in relation to the time of drug administration if serial sampling of a patient is required. When properly undertaken, drug monitoring is 90% accurate.

TOXIC CHEMICAL EXPOSURE

In our daily lives we are continually exposed to potentially toxic chemicals: paints, varnishes, disinfectants, polishes, deodorants, glues, pesticides to list but a few. Doctors are becoming increasingly aware that exposure to these substances can cause disease, disability, and in some cases, death. Deleterious effects are more likely after prolonged exposure, but brief contact can also cause unpleasant and even dangerous symptoms.

It is possible to test an individual's blood (see Chapter 2) for trace amounts of many chemicals. This information, when added to the patient's signs and symptoms may account for previously unexplainable disease. There are many different sorts of blood screening tests currently available, including:

- **General volatile screening test:** detects 12 organic chemicals

- **Chlorinated pesticide screening test:** detects 19 pesticides

- **Chlorinated phenols screening test:** detects polychlorinated biphenyls, and some fungicides and defoliants

- **Phenoxy acid screening test:** detects herbicides

- **Cholinesterase test:** measuring cholinesterase will detect a certain organic phosphate insecticide and certain herbicides.

It is not normal for any amount of a toxic chemical to be found in the blood. The problem is that so many people have been exposed to potentially dangerous chemicals that it is now usual, if not normal, for traces to be found. This is taken into account when 'normal' values are decided upon. However, the significance of any test result therefore depends entirely on the doctor's interpretation. Subjective decisions can be open to misuse — we have already seen in this country how the government applies different 'normal' values for radiation exposure, according to what is politically expedient, rather than what is necessarily medically safe.

CONCLUSION

With increasing drug use and abuse, and widespread exposure to a variety of potentially toxic chemicals, toxicology has developed rapidly. There are now simple, quick and reliable methods of testing for poisoning, and for establishing the cause of the observed symptoms and signs.

CANCER

Cancer is not one disease, but many. They have in common the way they grow, spread and behave. Certain cells suddenly lose their ability to respond to the normal control mechanisms of the body. They therefore divide rapidly, forming tumours. Tumours are often categorized as benign or malignant.

Benign: in which the cells tend to look normal and remain localised. If they do cause trouble it is because, for example, a tumour is pressing against an organ. These tumours are relatively easy to treat.

Malignant: these tumours look very different from the cells from which they were derived. They are not localised and have the capacity to invade and destroy the surrounding tissue, eventually spreading throughout the body. It is this mobility that makes malignant tumours so difficult to treat.

A better perspective however, would be to view benign/malignant as a sort of spectrum, with totally benign growths at one end such as lipoma; potentially malignant growth in the middle such as cystic fibroma; slow growing cancer about three quarters of the way along; and very malignant tumours with early spread at the other end.

Despite the fact that in the UK cancer is the second leading cause of death in both adults and children, doctors have not yet been able to find a definitive, or even consistently reliable test for early cancer detection. Screening for hidden cancers has also not been terribly successful. Even where there are screening programmes, as for breast and cervical cancer, controversy about their value is rife (see Chapter 6).

Most people who have cancer will have gone to their GP because they have felt unwell, or noticed particular symptoms such as a lump. Other cancers are picked up during routine examinations for other disorders. Because the symptoms may be vague, or similar to less dangerous conditions, there is a risk that the GP will miss the cancer; it will then remain undetected until it has reached a stage that is easily diagnosable — but often untreatable.

Even if the doctor suspects cancer, (s)he may avoid discussing this with you until some confirmatory tests have been performed. This evasion is usually well meant — there is a great deal of fear associated with cancer, and until a doctor is sure that a patient does have it, (s)he may be reluctant to generate unnecessary anxiety. Unfortunately, this behaviour can unwittingly contribute to the very anxiety that (s)he is trying to avoid. If you are somebody who prefers to know what is going on with your health it is worth questioning your doctor(s) at all stages of the diagnosis — asking them for all the information they have, including their uncertainties and possible alternative diagnoses.

In the event of cancer having been diagnosed it is vitally important that you realize your right to a second opinion. Cancer diagnosis is fraught with uncertainty, and there is a small chance that the original diagnosis is wrong. The same applies for the treatment you are offered. There are now many different forms of treatment, and before you submit to anything be sure you know what all the alternatives are. More and more research is showing that the most important factor in the success of any treatment is that the patient believes in it, and agrees to participate.

So, what are the diagnostic techniques employed to detect cancer? They vary according to

- the stage at which the cancer has been presented to the doctor

- the facilities available to the hospital or clinic undertaking the tests

- the location of the cancer.

By taking an accurate detailed history, feeling (palpation), listening with a stethoscope, and testing the body's functions (ie testing reflexes) a physician will gain enough information to form a diagnosis. Tests are then ordered to confirm that diagnosis. The following are the usual tests for cancer. More details of each test and how it is performed are given in Chapter 2.

BLOOD TESTS

There are an enormous range of tests that can be performed on a sample of your blood to indicate the presence of cancer in specific organs. However, they vary greatly in their specificity and levels of accuracy — a positive result may be due to the presence of a variety of conditions, not just cancer. Other diagnostic tests inevitably have to be ordered to eliminate these other possibilities.

RADIOGRAPHY

X-rays have played an extremely important part in the diagnosis of cancer — tumours can often be seen quite clearly, even when they are very small. Other techniques are now taking over, but for many years X-ray was the only imaging technique available.

Plain X-rays, or X-rays using contrast material to highlight certain organs are used. If required, the contrast media may be injected, taken by mouth or by an enema, depending on the organ to be investigated. For example, to outline the gullet, stomach, and upper part of the intestines you will be asked to partake of a 'barium meal' (a drink containing barium); whereas to outline the colon and rectum a barium enema is performed. Whatever the contrast material, there will be a certain amount of preparation. This varies from hospital to hospital, but your doctor should explain what will be required of you. For example, a special diet is recommended for several days prior to a barium enema; and for an X-ray of the lymph glands, contrast media is injected into the webs between the toes through two small incisions. This requires an overnight stay in hospital and the X-ray is then performed the following day. As the dye stays in the abdominal nodes for several months, regular abdominal X-rays are normally carried out without the need for further injections.

Contrast media are also commonly used to outline the kidneys, ureters and the bladder; the lymph glands; gall bladder; arteries and veins; and the spinal cord.

As with all tests you should ask why the test is being done, what the procedure will be, whether there are any after- or side-effects you should know about.

CT SCANS

CT scans are used to view the whole body and the brain. CT scans are useful for the examination of very small or indistinct structures. As with X-rays, special preparation is necessary prior to a CT scan; your doctor should explain what you must, or must not do.

NUCLEAR SCANNING

For all radioisotope scans, the isotope is injected, usually into a vein in your arm. This sort of scan is most commonly used to look at bone and the liver, although the gall bladder, lung, thyroid and kidney are also viewed by this technique.

ULTRASOUND

In the diagnosis of cancer, ultrasound is most commonly used to view the abdomen and pelvis. No special preparation is required, although if it is the gall bladder that is being examined, you will be asked not to eat anything for six hours beforehand. If it is the abdomen and pelvis, you will be asked to come for the test with a full bladder.

BIOPSY

If cancer is suspected, a biopsy will almost always be taken. All biopsies carry a small risk of complications such as infection or bruising and you should discuss with your doctor how these will affect you. The tissue removed by biopsy is, after being specially prepared, examined under a microscope. The cancer cells can then be identified, if present. But even biopsy may not give a clear answer as some cancers are difficult to detect, so a repeat biopsy may be taken to confirm the original diagnosis.

ENDOSCOPY

Scoping techniques are used to directly investigate certain organs for cancer — commonly, the rectum, colon, gullet, stomach, duodenum, gall bladder, pancreas and lungs.

CERVICAL SMEAR

See Chapter 6 for details.

DILATION AND CURETTAGE

See Chapter 6 for details.

SELF-EXAMINATION

These include:

- digital rectal examination

- breast self-examination

- testicle self-examination

- surveying one's skin and body for unusual markings, blemishes, and swellings.

These are all valuable cancer screening tests if you seek professional advice regarding any observed changes.

CONCLUSION

Most of the high technology diagnostic techniques are being used in the detection of cancer. Consequently diagnosis is being made at an earlier and earlier stage, which in turn improves the chances of successful treatment. In addition, improvements are being made in the screening programmes currently available, which should lead to even earlier detection of cancer.

EPILEPSY

Epilepsy is a symptom, not a disease. It is caused by sudden disturbances in the normal functioning of the brain. The word epilepsy is derived from the Greek, *epilambaneia*, which means 'to be seized by forces from without' — which was how fits and seizures were first characterized. There are many different types of fits and seizes and their incidence varies between individuals. The sort of fits people generally associate with epilepsy — unconsciousness followed by convulsion, and frothing at the mouth — are actually only suffered by a small number of individuals. Some epileptics merely stare vacantly for a second or two as they momentarily lose consciousness, others may only have convulsions in one part of their body.

The causes of the brain disturbances remain unclear and usually incurable. Treatment generally consists of controlling the seizures with the help of powerful drugs. Medication has, however, enabled the majority of epileptics to enjoy a relatively normal existence.

When presented with a patient complaining of seizures, it is vital that the doctor establishes definitively whether or not epilepsy is the right diagnosis. A mistaken diagnosis subjects the individual unnecessarily not only to medication with serious side effects, but also to disqualification from holding a driving licence and even the possible loss of employment — since ill-founded prejudice against people with epilepsy still prevails.

Once epilepsy is diagnosed, the doctor must then determine which type(s) of epilepsy the patient has. An incorrect seizure diagnosis can result in medication being prescribed that will not control the seizure and that may cause serious side effects.

If you have had one or more fits, your GP will, after an initial consultation with you about your symptoms, medical history and so on, refer you to a neurologist at your nearest hospital. You will be seen by the neurologist on an out-patient basis, and your appointment will take the following form:

THE INTERVIEW

At this initial interview the neurologist will want to establish the facts of your case. (S)he will ask you about your seizure(s).

● the symptoms preceding it

● what, if anything, seemed to bring it on

● when it occurred

● what happened during the seizure — the doctor usually asks for an eye witness account, since you may have been unconscious at the time

If you have experienced any strange hallucinations or deja vu (feeling that you have already experienced a present situation), you should mention this to the doctor. Many people omit to do so for fear of being diagnosed mentally ill, or because they seem irrelevant. In fact they provide important information about the sort of seizure you have had.

You will be asked about your previous medical history, for example, whether you have had any

● faints, convulsion or losses of memory or strange feeling states in the past

● major illnesses or accidents — for example, head injuries can bring on epilepsy.

Your family's medical history is also very important. Heredity does seem to play a part in epilepsy, so your neurologist will want to know if anyone in your family has had epilepsy or related disorders.

Finally the neurologist will ask you about general aspects of your life: your job, whether you drive, what sports you play, whether you smoke, drink, take drugs and so on.

This interview is your first opportunity to ask about epilepsy, and the neurologist should take time to answer any questions you may have.

In cases where the suspected epileptic is a newborn baby, the parents' medical histories and the history of the pregnancy and birth are all that the doctor has to go on. (S)he is therefore forced to rely heavily on physical examination and laboratory investigations for a diagnosis.

THE PHYSICAL EXAMINATION

After the interview, you will be asked to undress to your underwear in order for the neurologist to perform a physical examination. This will take between 15 to 20 minutes and will include the following:

- assessment of your general appearance

- examination of your skull for any unusual variation in contour

- examination of your limbs for

    - lack of symmetry
    - blemishes suggestive an organic disorder

- taking your pulse or blood pressure

- feeling your abdomen for the presence of any enlarged organs, and for women, a breast examination for cysts or tumours

- examination of the eyes, with an ophthalmoscope, for optic nerve damage

- testing your reflexes

    - knee jerk response to hitting your knee with a hammer

- response to having the soles of your feet stroked by the hammer (normally the big toe flexes downwards)

- **testing your grip for any muscular weakness**

- **listening to the heart and lungs, using a stethoscope, for any unusual murmurs.**

By the end of this examination the neurologist will probably have made a tentative diagnosis, but will usually send you for a series of tests for confirmation, before discussing the results.

INVESTIGATIVE TECHNIQUES

Your age when epilepsy is first suspected plays a major role in deciding what tests, in addition to the physical examination, are appropriate for evaluating your condition. For example, a girl whose seizures start when she is ten will be subjected to fewer and less invasive tests than a woman whose seizures begin at 40. The young person very probably has epilepsy, if no other neurologic problems were found during the physical examination, whereas the woman is at high risk from a brain tumour or central nervous system infection, even if the neurological examination is normal.

Some of the tests available provide little information that will be useful in reaching a diagnosis or deciding on therapy, so discrimination on the part of the doctor is important in choosing the most appropriate tests. The most useful diagnostic tools in the investigation of epilepsy are still clinical history and physical examination.

The tests chosen will usually be performed on a separate visit to the hospital — shortly after the initial interview. The following are the tests that neurologists can currently select from (see Chapter 2 for details of techniques):

ELECTROENCEPHALOGRAPHY (EEG)

This is the study of electrical activity in the brain. An EEG examination is not painful and is performed by a specially trained technician while you are fully conscious, sitting on a chair or lying on a couch. The technician will first fit the electrodes to your scalp. You will be asked to put on a rubber cap and the electrodes will be pushed through slats in the cap and attached to your scalp, either by a special glue or with a plastic mount with a silver rod on top. At one end of the rod is a pad of cotton wool covered in lint soaked in saline solution. With the latter type of electrode, the wires that carry the electrical impulses from the brain to the EEG machine are attached to them with crocodile clips. Electrodes attached with glue already have a wire built into them.

You will probably have been asked to wash your hair thoroughly for the test, as grease interferes with the electrical signals emitted through the skull. You should also avoid using hair spray for the same reason.

The EEG machine is designed to exclude most extraneous electricity, but to ensure a greater accuracy, the test is performed in an insulated room to prevent interference from mains electricity, radios and so on. You will be asked to remain still so that electrical activity on the muscles does not drown out those of the brain. Because children often find this difficult the technician may administer a short-acting barbiturate to sedate the child. This will extend the test by several hours.

During the test you will first be asked to open and shut your eyes several times in order for the technician to observe the alteration of the alpha and beta rhythms. Then you will be asked to hyperventilate (breathing at an abnormally rapid rate while at rest) for up to three minutes, and to look at a stroboscope flashing at 1 to 60 cps. These are both effective means of releasing abnormal rhythms that otherwise might remain hidden. The technician will stop the examination if the EEG read-out suggests that you are on the verge of having a seizure. The whole test takes about 30 minutes. The EEG is interpreted by a specially trained neurologist.

If the doctor wants a more extended EEG, there are now miniature EEGs available that are battery operated and allow a 24 hour EEG record without imposing undue restrictions on the patient.

While EEG has been useful in diagnosing many neurologic problems, it has had most impact in the investigation of epilepsy. Patients with a structurally normal brain may have seizures, but the EEG will not be normal in most cases of epilepsy. Although an EEG cannot establish the cause of epilepsy, some patterns do limit the possible causes of the brain damage. There are no known risks to EEG and when properly performed it is 95% accurate in the diagnosis of epilepsy.

LUMBAR PUNCTURE AND EXAMINATION OF THE CEREBRO-SPINAL FLUID

Lumbar puncture has limited use in the investigation of epilepsy and in some cases can be dangerous. It should therefore not be used as a routine investigation. It is performed when there is suspicion of a central nervous system infection, and is helpful in investigating certain problems that may cause seizures.

RADIOGRAPHY

- X-rays of the skull are useful in providing evidence of certain conditions, including increased intracranial pressure, intracranial calcification, local erosion and hyperostosis. But on the whole they are of diagnostic value in only a relatively small proportion of epileptic patients.

- X-rays of the chest are usually taken to exclude a primary carcinoma of the lung which may have spread to the brain, causing epilepsy. There are also other pulmonary pathologies which can have a subsequent effect on the brain, that a chest X-ray can identify.

- Contrast materials may be injected into a major artery in order to investigate certain intracranial lesions associated with epilepsy, as well as investigating various possible causes of seizures.

CT SCAN

CT scanning has had an enormous impact on all of neurology, and where available, individuals with seizures of recent onset are examined with this technique. Pregnant women with no focal neurologic signs should not undergo CT scans. CT scans can display tumours and atrophic lesions which may be the cause of epilepsy.

AIR ENCEPHALOGRAPHY

This test is only used where CT scans are not available, since it provides much the same information as a CT scan but is far more unpleasant for the patient. First you undergo a lumbar puncture, after which a small quantity of air is introduced into the spinal canal through a hollow needle. The air moves up the spine to fill the hollows at the centre of the brain known as the ventricles. These stand out clearly when photographed, enabling a doctor to recognize any abnormalities in their size and shape. During the test you will feel as though your head is being blown up like a balloon and it may take a couple of days for the headache to go.

RADIOISOTOPIC SCANNING

This is widely used as a screening technique in patients suspected of having a cerebral tumour. Radioisotopic scanning is not as useful as CT scans in investigating the causes of epilepsy since it cannot detect atrophic lesions.

ULTRASONIC ECHOENCEPHALOGRAPHY

This investigation is to look at structural changes in the brain. Although it is safe and painless it lacks the accuracy of CT and radioisotopic scan, and with their wider availability, its use is diminishing.

BIOCHEMICAL INVESTIGATIONS

You will be asked for samples of blood and urine for laboratory analysis. Many biochemical analyses can be performed on the samples and can provide valuable information in the diagnosis of epilepsy. Tests on the samples include:

- Serological tests for syphilis,

- Prolonged fasting blood glucose estimations,

- Tolbutamide tolerance tests or plasma insulin assays

- Estimations of serum calcium and blood urea.

The doctor may also take a small piece of tissue from the wall of the rectum in order to confirm a diagnosis of tumerous sclerosis or neurofibromatosis.

CONCLUSIONS

Once epilepsy is diagnosed it can usually be treated to the extent that the sufferer can live a relatively unrestricted life.

HEART AND CIRCULATION

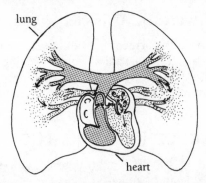

Pulmonary circulation 'Used' blood (dark shading) is pumped from the right ventricle through the pulmonary artery into the lungs. Capillaries in the lungs surround air sacs (alveoli) from which the blood easily absorbs oxygen and into which it expels carbon dioxide. The capillaries merge to become pulmonary veins. These carry the freshly oxygenated blood (light shading) into the left side of the heart.

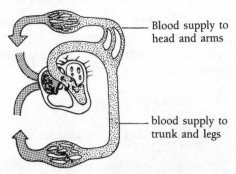

Systemic circulation The left ventrical is larger and more muscular than the right ventricle. This is because it has to pump oxygenated blood (light shading) to all parts of the body. The 'used' blood (dark shading) returns from body tissues to the heart through the veins.

Figure 10. Diagram showing the heart and circulatory system.

90

BLOOD PRESSURE

A check of the blood pressure is probably the most frequent test performed during any medical examination. It is also important from a screening point of view, for reasons described below.

The term blood pressure usually refers to the pressure of the blood in the arteries as opposed to the pressure in the veins. The pressure in the veins of the blood returning to the heart is a quite different and relatively unimportant pressure except in certain conditions (see below), whereas a persistently raised pressure in the arteries can cause irreversible damage.

ARTERIAL PRESSURE

The arterial blood pressure is affected by a number of factors:

- strength of each heartbeat

- elasticity of the walls of the artery

- amount of blood flowing

- thickness of the blood

- amount of certain hormones and enzymes (e.g. adrenaline) in the blood

- functioning of the sympathetic nervous system (the part of the nervous system not under voluntary control).

Through these mechanisms the blood pressure will also vary according to posture, stressful situations and other external stimuli.

The blood pressure is normally expressed as two figures (e.g. 120/80). This is because the blood pressure varies throughout each heartbeat cycle, reaching its peak when the main chambers of the heart contract, and its lowest point as they relax. The contraction phase of the heart is known as a systole and the relaxation as diastole, and the blood pressure is therefore known as the systolic pressure, (which is the figure on the left) and the diastolic

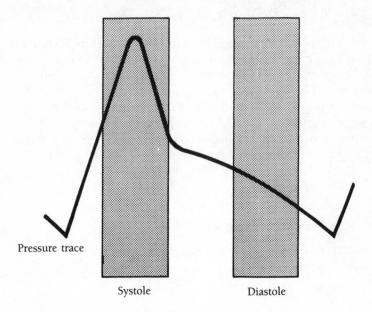

Figure 11. A pulse wave.

pressure (which is the figure on the right).

In order to measure the blood pressure an inflatable cuff is wrapped round a limb (usually the upper arm) and blown up to a point where the artery is compressed and closed. The pressure is then slowly reduced whilst a stethoscope is applied over the artery beyond the cuff. When a point is reached that the systolic pressure is sufficient to open the artery with each beat, a regular beating is heard through the stethoscope as the artery walls collapse between each contraction, causing a slapping sound. As the pressure is further released, there comes a point where the artery remains permanently open, which is the diastolic pressure, and the sound is therefore no longer heard.

Sometimes an estimation of blood pressure is taken by feeling the pulse rather than listening. When the cuff is inflated above the systolic pressure the pulse at the wrist disappears, but will reappear as the pressure is reduced when the systolic pressure is reached. But this method cannot give an indication of diastolic pressure.

Recently, electronic blood pressure machines have been developed which incorporate a small microphone in the cuff. These detect the start and end of the noise, and can therefore translate the pressure to a direct digital reading. These are therefore suitable for home use by patients, though accuracy can be affected if the microphone is not placed directly over the artery, and even when correctly used are not as accurate as an experienced clinician.

Blood pressure varies with posture and with stress and several readings may be taken during the course of an examination, in both the sitting and lying position. Patients are often anxious about visiting the doctor, and the anxiety may display itself in a falsely raised reading. For this reason many doctors will take several measurements of the blood pressure before deciding whether this truly represents an abnormal result, or even occasionally ask the patient or relative to take blood pressure at home. Very occasionally a twenty-four hour recording can be taken, where a small device repeatedly measures the patient's blood pressure during the day and night and automatically records this on to a tape. This can very occasionally be useful in diagnosing intermittent or stress induced hypertension.

VENOUS PRESSURE

The pressure of blood in the veins can be measured directly using a small tube on a needle placed directly into the vein. These tests can show some obstruction within the heart itself, or increase in blood volume during transfusions, but is not often used.

PULMONARY ARTERY PRESSURE

The pulmonary artery takes blood from the heart to the lungs, and is therefore not immediately accessible for measurement of pressure of blood within it. To perform this test a tube with a small balloon on the end is inserted through a vein and passed through the heart (using the balloon as a method of propulsion through the Chambers) until the tip of the tube is in the pulmonary artery. The pressure of blood can then be measured at the other end of the tube. However this is considered by many as an extremely dangerous test and in most instances offers no real benefit to the patient. Sometimes this test is performed on patients who are receiving intravenous fluids, to ensure that they are not overloaded, but it would seem that simple tests with venous blood pressure offer satisfactory monitoring in this situation.

RAISED ARTERIAL BLOOD PRESSURE

Raised blood pressure of itself can be an indication of an under-lying condition and therefore further tests are usually carried out if an abnormally high reading is found. Blood pressure may be raised without other conditions (essential hypertension) and this condition exists in approximately one person in ten, with increasing frequency above middle age. Other conditions which can cause raised blood pressure are:

- Kidney disease

- Thyroid or other hormone disease

- Obesity

- Heart or lung disease

- Pregnancy

Further tests (see Chapter 2) can reveal the presence of these problems.

NORMAL VALUE FOR BLOOD PRESSURE

The usual figure accepted for arterial blood pressure is 120/80 (that is the systolic pressure of 120mm of mercury and a diastolic pressure of 80mm of mercury). But as we get older the arteries lose their elasticity, and the blood pressure therefore naturally rises. Diastolic pressure is the greater indication of future problems, as this represents the persistent pressure rather than the inter-mittent systolic pressure. In general a diastolic pressure over 95mm of mercury is considered to be an indication of hypertension, though obviously one would be more concerned with this level in a twenty-five year old than in a sixty year old. One patient in five who is found to have a raised pressure will have a secondary cause which further tests will show.

LOW BLOOD PRESSURE

This most commonly occurs when moving from a lying or sitting to a standing position (usually in the elderly). It can also be caused by the following:

- drugs used to treat blood pressure (including diuretics)

- tranquillizers

- shock or severe blood loss.

SCREENING FOR RAISED BLOOD PRESSURE

Regular checks of blood pressure for all the adult population are important for the following reasons:

- Raised blood pressure may, of itself, not produce symptoms which suggest that the patient should seek advice.

- Persistently raised blood pressure may produce irreversible damage, which may not become apparent until the condition is life-threatening.

- Cardiovascular disease is the major cause of premature death in the UK and raised blood pressure is one factor predisposing to its development.

- The test is without risk, cheap, and painless.

ELECTROCARDIOGRAM

The most well known technical test to ascertain the function of the heart and circulatory system is the Electrocardiogram or ECG (sometimes abbreviated to EKG in view of the original German spelling). However, this only views the function of the heart in a limited sense, and gives no information regarding the state of the arteries in other parts of the system. To test these, Angiography is used, a form of X-rays using injected dyes, (see p 99).

Recent developments of these basic techniques allow more

sophisticated analysis of function, and the response of the system to emotional and physical stress.

The basic ECG indicates the activity of the electrical currents generated by the heart muscle which govern the expansion and contraction of the four main chambers. Electrodes are placed on the wrists and ankles, and eight further electrodes are attached to the chest, from the centre in a carefully positioned row under the left armpit. These electrodes are all simple metal pads designed to pick up tiny currents generated by the heart. They do not give out any current and the test therefore produces no sensation to the patient.

The twelve electrodes are connected to the machine which then examines, amplifies and records the electrical activity under each, or between a pair of electrodes. A standard set of recordings is obtained in this way. The recording is made onto a strip of paper, and shown on a screen. Switching between the various electrodes or 'leads' is automatic in modern machines, but is sometimes controlled manually.

The final record is a series of recordings which each shows a different electrical 'view' of the heart (Figure 12). From this apparently meaningless squiggle it is possible for the experienced practitioner to diagnose a number of heart problems:

- whether there is any damage to the heart muscle (as occurs in heart attack or coronary)

- whether the rhythm of the heart is normal and the contractions of the chambers are synchronised

- if there is any enlargement of a chamber (which can develop with raised blood pressure)

- if there is serious narrowing of the coronary arteries which supply blood to the heart (in angina).

Each peak on the recording corresponds to a particular activity in the heart. The P-wave shows the contraction of the atria, or the two small chambers of the heart, and R-wave indicates the contraction of the ventricles, the large chambers which propel blood around the body. The T-wave shows the depolarization (or

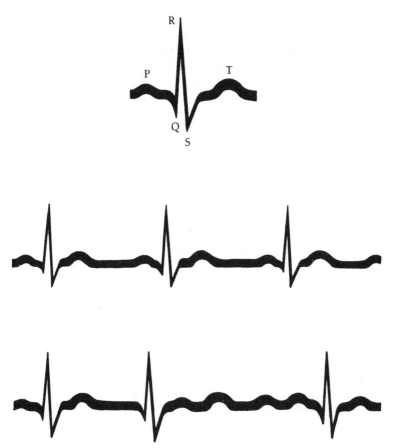

Figure 12. A ECG trace showing a normal complex (top), a normal series of complexes showing a normal rhythm (middle), and a trace showing an abnormal rhythm where the P waves are not synchronized with the QRS waves (atrial fibrillation).

release of electrical charge) of the whole of the heart preparatory to another cycle of contraction. Figure 12 shows a simple example of an abnormal ECG in that there is not the close association of one P-wave to each R-wave, but several unconnected P-waves. In this case the patient has atrial fibrillation, where the small chambers are contracting 'out of synch' with the larger ventricles.

The basic ECG is a relatively old test and there are now modern refinements to it:

THE 24 HOUR ECG

This test is designed to pick up abnormalities which are intermittent — particularly abnormal rhythms. The ECG recorder is portable, and worn constantly by the patient, and a small attached tape recorder keeps a constant record of his heart's activity. Sometimes a patient may also be asked to keep a separate record of particular activities during the day, such as physical or emotional stress, sleep, eating etc. When the tape is subsequently fed through a computer intermittent abnormalities will be revealed, and it may be possible to associate these with activity.

THE EXERCISE ECG

If a patient is suspected of having a degree of narrowing of the coronary arteries which does not show up on the normal ECG he may undergo an exercise or stress ECG. In this the leads remain attached and the recorder is left running whilst the patient undergoes exercise — either a treadmill, exercise bike, or even just up and down two steps constantly. The ECG will record the expected increase in heart rate, but will also show if the supply of oxygen to the heart becomes reduced — which reflects a poor blood supply. This test does have its limitations, firstly in that it is not without risk in a patient with a severe restriction of blood supply, and some normal patients show abnormalities on the exercise ECG which can lead to unwarranted concern.

THE ECHOCARDIOGRAM

This is unrelated to the ECG, but is sometimes used in conjunction with it. It is an ultrasound examination of the heart, whereby sound waves are sent into the heart from the body surface via a transducer and are reflected by the various surfaces. A picture of the heart in action is thus obtained and displayed on a screen, showing the size, action and efficiency of the chambers, and the function of the various valves.

USE OF THE ECG

Apart from the use in the conditions mentioned, the ECG is frequently used in health screening examinations. This has led to the idea that in some way the ECG is predictive, and that a normal ECG can be taken as reassurance that no heart disease will develop. Unfortunately, many heart problems — including serious ones — can develop rapidly and with no warning. The ECG is not a crystal ball.

ANGIOGRAPHY

This examination of the circulatory system, also called arteriography, is a form of X-ray examination to determine the state of the arteries. A dye, which is opaque to X-rays, and therefore shows up on X-ray photographs, is injected into an artery and allowed to circulate. X-rays will show any local narrowing or expansion of an artery. The most common sites for angiography are:

CAROTID ANGIOGRAPHY

In this the dye is injected into the carotid artery in the neck, which supplies blood to the brain. Any obstruction from a blood clot, or bleeding point will be shown (as in a stroke).

CORONARY ANGIOGRAPHY

Some patients with angina have localised narrowing of the coronary arteries around the heart, and surgery to by-pass the obstruction may be possible. In order to discover whether they are suitable an angiogram of the arteries is essential. In this a small tube, or catheter, is inserted into the artery in the arm and fed up, using guidance by X-rays, until it is positioned at the entrance to the coronary arteries at the top of the heart. When dye is injected it flows down the coronary arteries and displays their outline, showing any local narrowing that the surgeon must by-pass.

FEMORAL ANGIOGRAPHY

Some patients develop narrowing of the arteries in the legs, leading to pain on walking. This too can be surgically by-passed if the obstruction is over a short length, and can be shown by X-rays after dye is injected into the femoral artery in the thigh.

VENOGRAPHY

Using similar techniques to those in angiography, it is possible to show the outline of veins on X-rays. This test may be used when there is clinical suggestion of an obstruction or blood clot in the vein.

BLOOD TESTS IN HEART DISEASE

BLOOD TESTS

After a heart attack or coronary, where some of the heart muscle has been deprived of oxygen and therefore dies, there is a rise in some of the chemicals — particularly creatinine phosphokinase, or CPK — which the muscle produces. Estimation of the CPK and other enzyme levels can thus act as confirmation of a heart attack.

BLOOD LIPOPROTEIN LEVELS (CHOLESTEROL)

Some patients have an inborn alteration in the way their body uses fats — both fats in the diet and those produced by the body — and a proportion of them develop early arteriosclerosis or narrowing of the arteries. This can lead to premature heart or circulatory disease.

Fat in the blood combines with protein to form lipoproteins, and these are of various sorts, classified according to their weight or density. It seems that high levels of Low Density Lipoproteins (LDL) predispose to early disease whereas an increased concentration High Density Lipoproteins offers protection against arteriosclerosis.

From this it will be clear that a simple estimation of the total fat level in the blood is not sufficient on its own to identify those at risk. This basic test is used as a screening method, and patients displaying an increase of the total fat level will go on to have further tests to show which lipoproteins are specifically raised. Not only is this essential to discover whether treatment is necessary, but also what treatment should be used (diet, drugs or both).

SCREENING FOR HEART AND CIRCULATORY DISEASE

Disease of the heart and circulation accounts for 51% of deaths in the UK. Often this is sudden, premature, and the conditions leading to it have been unknown to the patient. Adequate screening could reduce this toll. Four factors are known to influence the development of diseases of the heart and circulation:

- Smoking

- Obesity

- Raised blood pressure

- Raised low density lipoproteins (as part of raised total blood fat)

Clearly patients know and can control (to some extent!) the first two factors. The others are symptomless, but easy and cheap to detect. In view of the prevalence and importance of this group of diseases there is considerable support for the idea that all the population, and particularly those with a family history of heart disease, should be checked for these conditions.

METABOLIC AND ENDOCRINE DISORDERS

'Metabolism' is the sum of all the chemical and physical changes taking place within our bodies to ensure continued growth and functioning. The 'endocrine system' masterminds healthy metabolic functioning. All major biological events in our life are controlled by the endocrine system, which is made up of glands that secrete hormones into the blood stream in order that they can travel to the organs they act on. There is also a profound relationship between the endocrine system and the central nervous system. The glands composing the endocrine system include the

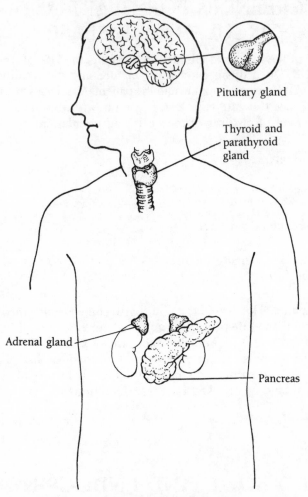

Figure 13. Diagram showing the hormone-producing glands.

adrenals, pancreas, pineal, pituitary, parathyroids, thyroid, testes (in men) and the ovaries (in women).

BASAL METABOLIC RATE (BMR)

The BMR can be used to measure general metabolic functioning, and to investigate suspected endocrine disease. BMR is primarily a measure of thyroid function and to some extent has been superseded by other more accurate tests. At best, BMR is only about 60% accurate.

You are required to fast beforehand and to be as relaxed as possible during the test. You may therefore be asked to lie, undisturbed, in a darkened room for an hour or so before the test. You are then asked to breathe into a machine that measures the body's oxygen consumption and the calories expended while at rest. The test takes about 20 minutes to perform, during which time your movements are necessarily restricted — as they may affect the results. Normal values for you are calculated according to your age, height and weight. An elevated value may indicate hyperthyroidism, acromegaly, diabetes insipidus, Cushing's disease, leukemia, pulmonary and cardiovascular disease, acidosis — and anxiety! Hypothyroidism is indicated when the BMR is lower than normal.

BMR is usually performed on an in- or out-patient basis at hospital. The only risk is infection from an unsterilised machine, and the only discomfort is that of being restricted for a longish period of time.

METABOLIC SCREENING

The purpose of metabolic screening is to identify abnormal compounds or abnormal amounts of metabolites in the body fluids of anyone suspected of having an inherited metabolic disorder. Your GP will have referred you or your child for tests. The samples of body fluids taken will be analysed at a hospital laboratory.

The most commonly used sample for metabolic screening is an accurately timed and measured urine sample (see Chapter 2). Most pathological compounds can be found in the urine in larger amounts, given the volume of urine, than in blood or plasma. Timed urine samples are used because they provide information on the amount of metabolites produced in a given period. Twenty-four hour collections reduce the effect of the normal daily variations in the excretion of metabolites. This may not be possible with very young or severely retarded children — where four eight-hour samples may have to suffice.

There are certain tests that can only be performed with plasma or serum. You will be told what sample the laboratory requires from you.

DIAGNOSTIC TESTS FOR ENDOCRINE FUNCTION AND DISEASE

Diagnosis here mostly relies on analysis of samples of blood or urine. Before a sample is taken, you may have been asked to take or have injected, certain substances. These compounds have known properties in relation to the functioning of the gland under investigation. Your body's response to the drug will give the doctor a good indication of what is wrong with you.

Many of the tests involve *Radioimmunoassay* — which is a technique of using radioactive tracers to determine the levels of particular antibodies in the blood. For example, it is possible to 'label' the hormone insulin. In some diabetic patients insulin provokes the formation of anti-insulin antibodies, which combine with the insulin. After injection of the tracer insulin, samples of the patient's blood are analysed by electrophoresis or chromatography and the antibody components of the blood are tested for the presence of radioactivity.

ADRENAL GLANDS

The main hormone secreted by the adrenal glands is a glucocorticoid, a substance which has anti-inflammatory and metabolic activity, called Cortisol (hydrocortisone). Tests of adrenal functioning or disease often rely on measuring this hormone.

Tests of adrenal function include:

THE THORN TEST (adrenal function eosinophil count test)

ACTH (ACTH is secreted by the pituitary and causes the adrenal gland to secrete cortisol) is injected and its effect on certain white blood cells (eosinophils) is noted. Normally, cortisol would be produced and would decrease the number of eosinophils by half within four hours. If this does not happen the adrenal gland is not functioning as it should.

Cortisol testing is also used to detect congenital adrenal disease in a newborn baby. Cortisol measurements can be made from amniotic fluid (amniocentesis). In addition the values can be used as a means of evaluating the maturity and effectiveness of the lungs of a developing foetus.

URINE TESTS

Some urine tests are:

urine testing for pregnanetriol   a hormone metabolic product which is used as a confirmatory criterion for adrenal gland pathology and ovary tumour

urinary 17-ketosteroids   measurement of adrenal activity. This test is no longer considered the most reliable measurement of adrenal activity

urinary 17-hydroxycorticosteroids   measures how much cortisol the adrenals are secreting.

When adrenal disease is suspected (such as organically caused depression, Cushing's syndrome and tumours), a doctor will usually perform an *adrenal suppression test.* You will be given a synthetic glucocorticoid and blood and urine samples taken in order to measure cortisol levels. The adrenal glands normally produce the greatest amount of cortisol in the early morning and the smallest amount in the evening. Shift work can reverse this so it is important for the doctor to know your active and sleeping times. Emotions also have a strong influence on the adrenal gland so the doctor will want to establish your mental state.

Other diagnostic techniques include:

the ACTH stimulation test.   This is less accurate than the adrenal suppression test. ACTH is injected — if there is no increase in plasma cortisol, an adrenal tumour is indicated.

the Metyrapone test.   You are given the drug metyrapone, which prevents direct cortisol production to determine if ACTH will stimulate the adrenals. The drug is usually given at midnight, and cortisol levels are measured the next morning. Normally, the drug-induced reduction in cortisol will cause the body's ACTH to stimulate cortisol production; failure to produce cortisol indicates that the problem lies within the pituitary gland rather than in the adrenals. Birth control pills and other oestrogens can give false positive results. A new chemical Cosyntropin, which acts like ACTH is beginning to be used instead of ACTH because it requires less time, and does not provoke the allergic reaction that sometimes comes from pure ACTH.

CT Scan for detecting tumours

PANCREAS

The pancreas secretes the following hormones:

- insulin: involved in blood sugar and carbohydrate metabolism

- glucagon: helps control the amount of insulin in the body

It also makes and gives off other products, primarily enzymes, that aid in food digestion:

- amylase

- lipase

- trypsin

- chymotrypsin

- bicarbonate

DIAGNOSIS OF PANCREATIC DISORDERS

DIABETES MELLITUS

This is a disorder of carbohydrate metabolism in which sugars in the body are not oxidized to produce energy due to the lack of the hormone insulin. This is distinct from the rare condition diabetes insipidus — which is caused by deficiency of the pituitary hormone, vasopressin.

Diagnosis of diabetes depends on detecting the presence of abnormally high glucose levels in the blood and urine. There may be certain classic symptoms that will have brought the patient to the doctor — weight loss, increase in urine production, and abnormal thirst. But many patients are symptomless and high blood or urine glucose may only be noticed as part of a routine examination. Since abnormally high glucose levels do not necessarily mean diabetes — particularly if there are no other symptoms, an *oral glucose tolerance test* (OGTT) is performed. In order for this test to be conclusive you should have eaten a normal diet — containing at least 150g of carbohydrate — for three days before the test. Restriction of carbohydrates may lead to a sluggish insulin response and a false-positive result. There are also drugs which disturb carbohydrate tolerance, so you should tell the doctor of any medication you may be taking. Prolonged bed rest, fever or stress, trauma or surgery may also lead to a temporary deterioration in glucose tolerance, in which case, the test should be repeated later.

The test will be performed in the morning after an overnight fast of 10 to 12 hours, during which water may be drunk. You will be given glucose dissolved in water to drink. Blood samples (venous or capillary) are collected before you drink the glucose, and then at two hourly intervals thereafter. Urine samples are taken at the same time. The results will be made available very quickly. If you are a diabetic it is important to monitor your condition on a regular basis. Techniques include:

blood glucose monitoring: It is important for diabetics to maintain the level of blood glucose within a normal range. This requires regular monitoring. There are now a number of different blood monitoring kits on the market:

blood glucose testing strips: These strips contain chemicals which gradually change colour and darken in proportion to the amount of glucose in a drop of blood. Manufacturers instructions should be followed carefully. Diabetic clinics can supply you with testing strips, and they are also available on prescription.

To simplify pricking your finger there are now automatic finger prickers with a spring that does the pricking. They are designed to produce the smallest hole needed to obtain an adequate drop of blood. When pricking your finger, by whatever method, ensure that your hand is clean and dry, and that any antiseptic has been washed away, as this reacts with the strip. It is easier to get blood out of a warm finger, and be warned that a cold room or outside temperature may also cause low glucose results.

blood glucose meters: blood glucose monitoring strips can also be read by a meter that gives a digital display of the blood glucose level. This is useful for diabetics who are colour blind. As when reading the strip by eye, it is very important to follow the manufacturer's instructions about timing and test conditions.

Some hospitals and clinics have computers that will interpret results from certain meters to show, for example, your average pre-lunch glucose over the preceding month. Others perform a glycosylated haemoglobin A1 test which gives an indication of your average blood glucose level over a period of several weeks before the blood was taken. This test can assess the accuracy of your own finger prick blood tests. It is also useful for diabetics who rarely or never test their blood glucose level. Obviously the figure it gives is an average and may hide wild fluctuations over that period. Also the results can be affected if you are anaemic or have any condition in which the life of the red blood cells is shortened.

urine glucose tests: The kidneys help to maintain the normal blood glucose concentration by saving glucose from being excreted. However, glucose will be excreted in the urine when the blood glucose level rises above the kidney or renal threshold (which varies between individuals). The glucose concentration in a urine sample therefore represents how much above the renal threshold the blood glucose was during the time it took for the urine to collect in the bladder. Testing the urine for glucose is not as accurate as blood glucose tests, because they depend on each person's renal threshold, and only represent an average — depending on how long the urine has been collecting in the bladder. They are a useful indicator of general glucose control if your renal threshold is known. There are now many kits available on the market — remember to use manufacturer's instructions.

OTHER DISORDERS OF THE PANCREAS

These are often difficult to diagnose. Diseases include:

- acute and chronic pancreatitis

- stones

- cancer

- pancreatic insufficiency

The following techniques are used in diagnosis:

Blood Tests	most disorders
Abdominal Ultrasound	tumour, cancer, pancreatitis
Abdominal tap	pancreatitis
Endoscopy	cancer
CT scan	pancreatitis
X-ray (endoscopic retrograde cholangiopancreatogram)	pancreatic duct obstructions
Faeces examination	pancreatic insufficiency

PITUITARY GLAND

The pituitary is the master endocrine gland. It is made up of two lobes. The anterior lobe secretes the following hormones:

- thyroid-stimulating hormone (TSH)

- ACTH

- gonadotrophins

- growth hormone

- prolactin

- lipotrophin

- melanocyte-stimulating hormone

The secretion of all these hormones is regulated by specific hormone releasing factors, which are produced in the hypothalmus. The posterior lobe secretes the following hormones:

● vasopressin

● oxytocin

Most pituitary function tests do not directly measure the hormones given off by the pituitary gland; instead they are reflections of other gland and organ functions that are either activated or controlled by pituitary hormones. Tests include those for vasopressin, growth hormone, thyroid function, cortisol, prolactin, oestrogen, testis function and pregnancy.

Sometimes a combined *pituitary function test* is performed. This includes the simultaneous administration of thyrotophin-releasing hormone (TRH), LH releasing hormone (LHRH), and insulin-induced hypoglycaemia. The insulin-induced hypoglycaemia is used for investigating somatotrophin, prolactin, and corticotrophin secretion. The combined pituitary function should not be carried out on patients over 60 years old, or on patients with cardiovascular problems or a history of fits.

You will have to fast overnight, but are allowed free access to water. The test is done between 8 am and 10 am before breakfast. You should be asked to lie down and make yourself comfortable. A catheter is then inserted into a vein in your arm. After an initial rest period of half an hour, a basal blood sample is taken. Soluble insulin is then administered in a recommended dose for your body weight and medical condition. A blood sample is then taken every 15 minutes for the first hour and every 30 minutes after injection. You will experience some or all of the following symptoms during the test:

● sweating

● headaches

● raised blood-pressure

● increased heart rate

The hypoglycaemia lasts about 15 to 20 minutes after which you will feel very hungry and should be given a full breakfast.

The various blood-samples are then analysed and the concentrations of glucose and particular hormones are estimated.

A glucose tolerance test is used with patients with acromegaly (swelling of the feet, hands and face as a result of excessive production of the growth hormone as a result of a tumour in the anterior lobe). You will have to fast overnight and between 8 am and 10 am a basal blood sample is taken and 50g of glucose given orally. Blood samples are then taken every 30 minutes for two hours. Glucose and growth hormone concentrations are estimated in each sample. If the growth hormone has not been suppressed by the glucose, acromegaly is diagnosed.

Other blood tests for pituitary disease include:

- **testing for prolactin using a fasting morning blood sample**: higher than normal values may indicate a tumour of the pituitary

- **testing for progesterone**: low values may be due to pituitary disease (can be done on urine too)

- **testing serum osmolality (concentration of particles dissolved in a given quantity of blood serum)**: greater or less than normal values indicate disease

- **testing for testosterone**: less than normal values may mean pituitary disease

PARATHYROID GLANDS

The parathyroid glands are found within the thyroid gland, but are distinct from it. The hormones they produce control the body's calcium needs and use. One way of testing parathyroid function, and indeed investigating suspected abnormalities, is to measure the blood calcium in the serum from venous blood. It can also be measured in the urine, faeces and in the spinal fluid (see Chapter 2 for details). If correctly performed, the test is about 90% accurate in verifying the existence of numerous conditions.

THYROID

The thyroid gland is concerned with regulation of the metabolic rate by the secretion of two thyroid hormones — thyroxine (T4) and triodothyronine (T3), which are stimulated by thyroid stimulating hormone (TSH) from the pituitary gland and require trace amounts of iodine.

Originally the BMR was used to measure thyroid function, but it has now been overtaken by a selection of far more sophisticated tests that can be performed on venous blood samples from the patient.

The most common tests include:

- measuring T4 value in the serum

- measuring T3 uptake

- an FT1 (free thyroxine index — calculated by multiplying the T4 value by the uptake value)

- TSH estimation

Certain drugs can influence thyroid function tests, including:

- hormones (corticosteroids, oestrogens, progesterone, oral contraceptives)

- oral anticoagulants

- diphenylhydantoin

- large doses of aspirin

- antithyroid drugs

- sulphonamides

- lithium

- clofibrate

- recent radioactive scanning

More than one abnormal thyroid function test result must be obtained before thyroid dysfunction can be diagnosed, and where a patient has not got two more clinical signs of thyroid disease, the tests have no real significance. The tests are positive in less than half of 1% of those patients without signs and symptoms. Overall they have an 85% accuracy rate.

In order to establish whether the thyroid problems come from the pituitary rather than the thyroid itself, you may be asked to undergo the *thyroid stimulation test*. You are given TSH, then the physician observes its effect on the thyroid.

Other techniques used in diagnosing thyroid conditions include:

Biopsy   cancer, specific thyroid disease

Nuclear scan   cancer, specific thyroid disease

Ultrasound   cancer, tumour

TESTES

See Chapter 7.

OVARIES

See Chapter 6.

CONCLUSION

The effects of metabolic and endocrinal disorders are always profound. Fortunately there are reliable diagnostic and screening techniques available, and once the diagnosis has been confirmed, successful treatment of most disorders is possible.

RHEUMATIC DISORDERS

Rheumatic disorders include all diseases involving joints, tendons, muscles, ligaments, and associated structures. The most common of these disorders are osteoarthritis and rheumatoid arthritis. In Britain, 12% of all cases seen by GPs are due to rheumatic diseases, and the number of work days lost due to these complaints runs into many millions.

The causes of rheumatic disorders are varied: injury, infection, congenital and developmental problems, metabolic disorders, age, climate, obesity (in osteoarthritis), sex, heredity, and altered immunity (as in rheumatoid arthritis where the immune system appears to act against the affected joint); all these are implicated.

In order to investigate suspected rheumatic disorders there are a range of tests that can be employed. Whatever combination is used depends on which condition your doctor suspects is present. The most useful techniques are the analysis of synovial fluid and radiology. With all the following tests you should discuss the value of having them, the risks involved, and if you decide to go ahead, establish when the results will become available.

LABORATORY TESTS

BLOOD TESTS

The following tests may be performed on a sample of your blood:

haematological tests: These include:

- erythrocyte sedimentation rate, which is a good non-specific indicator of inflammation and infection, and

- a full blood count

biochemical tests: measurements of urea, electrolytes, calcium, inorganic phosphate, alkaline phosphatase, protein, protein electrophoresis, uric acid immunoglobins, liver function tests. The levels found provide valuable information on what condition is causing your symptoms.

autoantibodies tests: these are used for:

rheumatoid factor — the majority of sufferers of rheumatoid arthritis have an immunoglobulin antibody called rheumatoid factor (RH). The more RH detected in the blood, the greater the possibility that rheumatoid arthritis exists. However, other conditions (liver, lung and heart conditions, syphilis and some worm infestations) also increase RH levels, so further tests are needed to exclude them.

antinuclear antibodies — these antibodies are found most commonly in people with systemic lupus erythematosus (SLE), an inflammatory disease of connective tissue, although they may also be found in people who have relatives with SLE, but who do not themselves have the disease. As with tests for RH, this test is not very specific, and can only be used to confirm a diagnosis.

Both tests are useful in cases of suspected generalized rheumatic diseases.

URINALYSIS

(See Chapter 2 for details).

You may be asked to provide a mid-stream sample of urine (MSU), which will then be sent to a laboratory for microscopic examination of the sediment, and analysis of protein. Urinalysis is also useful of establishing any renal involvement in connective tissue disease, or renal toxicity in patients who are receiving drugs such as gold or penicillamine.

SYNOVIAL FLUID

Synovial fluid is found in all body joints. It helps lubricate the bone or cartilage surfaces. Analysis of synovial fluid is diagnostic for gout, septic arthritis, osteoarthritis, haemarthrosis and rheumatoid arthritis and in the differentiation of inflammatory from non-inflammatory arthropathies.

A sample is removed by aspiration (see Chapter 2 for details), usually from the knee joint. A local anaesthetic is used only if you already have an osteoarthritic joint, or can persuade the doctor that you are so nervous about the procedure that an anaesthetic is necessary! In most instances you will be asked to fast the night before and the morning of the test so as not to abnormally alter the sugar level in the synovial fluid. This is important as sugar levels is one of the things measured.

The fluid is examined immediately after withdrawal for its general appearance, since this changes if certain conditions are present — for example, it becomes more yellow or yellowish green

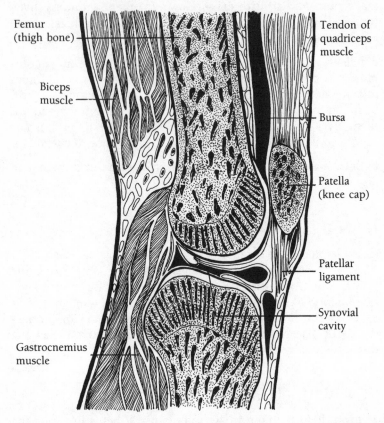

Figure 14. The structure of the knee, showing the synovial cavity.

and cloudy with arthritis. A series of tests are then performed on the fluid and it is examined microscopically.

The tests performed are from 20 to 65% accurate depending on the condition being investigated, but can differentiate between joint infection and other noninfectious conditions.

RADIOLOGICAL INVESTIGATIONS

X-rays (see Chapter 2 for details) of affected areas are routinely performed where rheumatic disease is suspected. An X-ray of the chest may also be performed because pulmonary cancer and TB may cause musculoskeletal symptoms, and respiratory and cardiovascular symptoms may occur as part of rheumatoid arthritis, seronegative arthritis and connective tissue disorders.

Radioisotope scanning is used, with a bone seeking isotope in order to detect certain bone abnormalities which do not show up on ordinary X-rays.

SYNOVIAL BIOPSY

Synovial biopsies can be formed in three different ways:

- needle biopsy under local anaesthetic — this is helpful in diagnosis of monoarthritis

- a biopsy can also be taken during arthroscopy (see below)

- open surgical biopsy under general anaesthetic — this is usually performed if TB is suspected.

The biopsy specimen is processed for histology, crystal examination, electron microscopy, and immunofluorescent studies.

ARTHROSCOPY

The interior of the knee joint is visualized via a rigid glass fibre arthroscope. Only a limited examination is possible under local anaesthetic; for a full examination general anaesthetic is required (see Chapter 2 for details of scoping procedures).

BONE BIOPSY

Under certain circumstances a biopsy specimen will be taken from some of your bone. Bone biopsies are most often performed to evaluate abnormal results from other tests — in particular X-rays. The specimen will be obtained either by a needle biopsy under local or general anaesthetic, or by an open biopsy under general anaesthetic. The biopsy site will probably be painful and tender for up to a week after the biopsy.

Muscle biopsies are sometimes also performed.

CONCLUSION

Rheumatic disorders are extremely common, particularly among the elderly. A variety of diagnostic techniques are available to help doctors determine the nature of the disorder. Their accuracy varies, and some techniques do carry with them certain risks. Because of this, and the limited treatment available to sufferers, patients should always discuss the value of any proposed technique before agreeing to undergo it.

ALLERGIES AND FOOD INTOLERANCE

In recent years there has been an increasing awareness of conditions which may be caused, at least in part, by the presence of allergies in the patient. Allergic diseases are extremely common. Estimates have been made that approximately one in five of the population has some form of allergy, though this may be only minor and cause mild irritation. However, allergic disease can cause severe conditions and the true incidence of allergic disease, including food intolerance, is unknown.

At present it is uncertain why there seems to be an increase in allergic disease this century. It may be that there is greater awareness of the problem, or it may be that our present day environment with its pollutants, food industry, and exposure to animal products lends itself to the creation of more allergic disease within us.

WHAT IS ALLERGY?

The word allergy is derived from the Greek and means simply 'an altered reaction'. In orthodox medicine it is usually confined to conditions which are produced within minutes of ingestion or contact (either through the skin or via the respiratory system) of an allergic substance. This immediate reaction is known as a type one allergy and covers rashes due to foods (strawberries and shellfish are common examples) as well as the immediate nasal discharge and sneezing brought on by contact with some dusts and pollens in certain individuals.

In addition to this type of reaction it is now becoming more accepted that other substances can cause delayed reactions, occurring maybe several hours after contact. This is particularly so in cases of food allergy. Indeed many workers believe the term allergy in these cases is a misnomer as the condition is more akin to an intolerance. With a strictly allergic reaction even the smallest amount of the substance can produce affects, but with delayed reactions the level has to go above a certain limit before symptoms are shown. It is better therefore to consider this an intolerance to more than a specific amount.

THE MECHANISMS OF ALLERGY

The reactions due to allergies are caused by four chemicals in the blood known as immunoglobins; these are known as IgE, IgG, IgA and IgM. A type one allergy is usually mediated by IgE, and an allergic individual can usually be detected by a raised level of IgE. However, IgE resides mainly in the skin and allergic reactions manifested via the skin therefore show a rise in IgE without necessarily a rise in the other immunoglobins. When an allergic response is initiated IgE causes the release, from specific cells in the skin, known as mast cells, of histamine which produces the allergic response.

IgG is mainly found in the serum, and IgA is mainly found in the intestines. IgM is in many tissues. It is IgA which possibly has a role to play in the mediation of type one food allergies, although it would seem that the mechanisms of other reactions to foods are yet to be understood.

MASKED ALLERGIES

As some allergic reactions can be delayed up to many hours it is sometimes difficult to identify a particular substance which is causing the sensitivity. Indeed if this is a commonly found item (i.e. a daily item in the diet) then persistent and chronic symptoms can develop without the patient being aware that this is due to an allergic response. Furthermore, if the item is identified and withdrawn then a period of hypersensitivity develops during which a small amount of the substance can produce dramatic and severe responses.

COMBINED ALLERGY

Some symptoms may be due to allergy to several different items, thus an allergic rhinitis may be due to dietary and inhaled allergens.

SUBSTANCES CAUSING ALLERGY

It is generally accepted that some of the following can and frequently do cause allergy:

● **Pollens, mould spores, other items of plant origin**

● **Dust (especially house dust), animal dander**

● **Alcohols, chemicals from industry, detergents, and fumes from combustible hydrocarbons (e.g. petrol fumes)**

● **Foods.**

Other substances are also implicated, but less accepted by the present orthodoxy. Identification of allergens can be extremely difficult and time consuming, especially as the tests for allergy are not as yet 100% reliable as the body's response to the allergen varies according to what it is.

CONDITIONS CAUSED BY ALLERGY

The symptoms caused by allergic disease can display the same features as a very large range of conditions. In addition they may be partially responsible in the cause of well recognized diseases.

Some conditions which may be caused by allergy are:

- Respiratory system: asthma, rhinitis, sinusitis.

- Migraine and other headaches.

- Psychological: mood swings, sleep disturbance, hyperactivity, learning disorders, depression and anxiety.

- Gastrointestinal system: abdominal distention, irritable bowel syndrome, spastic colon, possibly Crohn's disease and ulcerative colitis.

- Some arthritis, (not seropositive rheumatoid arthritis).

- Skin conditions: eczema, urticaria, possibly some psoriasis.

- Cardiovascular system: palpitations and abnormal heart rhythm.

- Endocrine system: premenstrual syndrome and menopausal complaints.

Obviously many of the above diseases may have purely physical causes rather than allergic, and it is difficult to differentiate between the two. Some important clues to allergy may be revealed in the history of the condition.

Other key features suggesting that a condition may be allergic in origin are:

- Symptoms which fluctuate and vary without any relation to any particular environmental factor.

- Weight fluctuations.

- Mental and psychological problems which are common in people with allergic disease. In particular they may suffer from excess fatigue which is inexplicable.

- Generalized aching in the joints and muscles which may

be a predominant or minor symptom.

- A particular craving for a specific food, or indeed a liking almost to the point of addiction, of a specific item (e.g. petrol fumes) which may be an indication that there is a sensitivity. Indeed there seems to be a close relationship between addiction and allergy.

DIAGNOSIS OF ALLERGY

Although there a number of tests available for detecting allergic reactions, none of these is 100% reliable, and sometimes it is possible to identify the particular agent from manipulation of the diet and the environment. Clearly if there is a type one allergic reaction, the item responsible can easily be identified, but if the reaction is delayed, this becomes more difficult. If a food is thought to be implicated, then exclusion of this food may well bring about a resolution, but often there is more than one food involved, and exclusion of them all can cause considerable dietary problems, especially in children. Testing by some method then becomes imperative.

TESTS FOR ALLERGY

These can be summarized under four headings:

- Tests based on skin reactions

- Tests based on blood reactions

- Tests based on dietary and environmental manipulation

- Test based on as yet unproven methods.

SKIN BASED TESTS

These are the prick, scratch and patch tests.

PRICK TEST

In this test a drop of a solution of the suspected substance is injected into the skin and a small blister is raised. The reaction of the skin after some minutes is estimated (as shown by the development of a weal and reddening around the point of injection) and the size of this area is thought to be an indicator of the severity of the allergy. Some patients reacted in a very severe manner to prick tests and this has therefore been superseded by:

SCRATCH TEST

In this test the skin is scratched through a drop of the suspected agent and a similar reaction to that of the prick test is noted.

PATCH TEST

This test is used mainly for items which can cause a contact allergy (i.e. a skin reaction when a substance comes into direct contact with the skin) and consists of a strip of adhesive material in which there are small cups. Into these cups are placed samples of potential allergens (an 'allergen' is a substance causing an allergic reaction) and the strip is then stuck to the back of the patient for forty-eight hours. A skin reaction under a particular cup indicates that this is a positive test.

All skin based tests are limited in that they are only useful for non-food allergens and are at best probably only 60% correct. In addition they are unpleasant in that there is some discomfort involved both in testing procedure and with the reaction afterwards. This makes these tests difficult for children.

BLOOD BASED TESTS

Two tests are available using samples of the patient's blood:

RAST TEST

This involves the radioactive labelling of allergens which are then mixed with the serum of the patient. Antibodies in the blood will attach themselves to the allergens and counting by radiographic means will estimate the amount of allergen present. Therefore this test can be used to show both a positive reaction and its degree of severity. The drawbacks of this test are that it is not widely available, expensive (approximately £7.50 per item tested), and is dependent on the skill of the operator.

CYTOTOXIC TEST

This involves the mixing of white cells from the patient's blood with the suspected allergen. Observation through a microscope will show degeneration of the white cells in a positive reaction. Unfortunately this test is even more operator dependent and has been discredited as inaccurate.

DIETARY TESTS

Dietary manipulation can be useful in food allergy, but obviously not in other allergies. These consist of:

EXCLUSION AND CHALLENGE TESTS

If the patient fasts for five days and then introduces one food item on alternate days, any reaction to a specific food can be identified.

ROTATION DIETS

These are not so time consuming or difficult, and consist of the consumption of particular groups of foods on different days, in order to ascertain the group responsible.

Clearly both of these approaches demand considerable will power and time. They may also be DANGEROUS WITHOUT SUPERVISION as deficiencies in essential items of diet may result. You should therefore consult your doctor or an allergy specialist if you want to try this method.

OTHER TESTS

There are a number of other tests, particularly in the unorthodox field which may be useful, but are not widely accepted at present as the mechanism is unclear. These include tests using the pulse, muscle power (applied kineseology) and electronic methods. Their full use has yet to be evaluated.

SCREENING FOR ALLERGY

Despite the apparently high incidence of allergic problems, widespread screening is not at the moment feasible in view of the lack of reliable and accepted tests, and the fact that allergic illness, whilst debilitating to the patient, is not often life-threatening (except for severe asthma). An experienced and broad-minded practitioner is usually able to realize that a patient's symptoms are due to an allergy and advise them accordingly.

SEXUALLY TRANSMITTED DISEASES (Venereal Disease)

Sexually transmitted diseases (STDs) are infectious diseases usually transmitted by sexual activity and include:

- Gonorrhea
- Nongonococcal urethritis
- Nonspecific vaginitis
- Trichomonal vaginitis
- Candida vaginitis
- Molluscum contagiosum
- Venereal warts
- Genital herpes

- Syphilis

- Scabies

- Pediculosis pubis

- Chancroid

- Lymphogranuloma venereum

- Granuloma inguinale

The number of reported cases in the UK has risen threefold in 15 years — with 600,000 new ones added each year. This may be a real increase, or the result of improvements in the service offered by clinics including their ability to trace sexual contacts so that more people are now seeking treatment. There are certainly more clinics specializing in the diagnosis and treatment of STDs than 15 years ago — 230 departments of genito-urinary medicine alone.

TESTING FOR STDs

There are some home tests for STDs, but there is no substitute for professional help should you have any cause for concern. In most incidences this means a visit to a STD clinic. GPs are generally not well equipped for accurate diagnosis of STDs, and will usually refer you to a specialist clinic anyway. Many people are reluctant to go to their GP — particularly if they are known to them socially — because of embarrassment and misplaced guilt. Since you do not need a referral, you can choose the clinic you prefer, even if it is not in your immediate area. Telephone numbers are in the phone book, but Citizens' Advice Bureaux and Family Planning Clinics also give addresses, as will your GP. Some clinics have an appointment system, others simply invite patients to walk in and be seen. Some run a combined system.

The stigma of having to visit an STD clinic has diminished in recent years. Staff no longer cast themselves as guardians of public morality and are generally helpful and supportive.

On arrival at the clinic you will be given a card with your name and a clinic number for future appointments. Most clinics have a record system separate from that of the main hospital to ensure confidentiality, and you do not have to give your address or telephone number if you do not want to. Your GP will only be informed of the diagnosis if you were referred to the clinic by them. Any inquiries, for example, from solicitors or doctors performing life assurance examinations, would not be answered unless the patient gives written permission. The police are never given information, even if the patient is a minor, unless the patient requests it.

Once registered, you will be interviewed by a doctor. (S)he will ask you questions about your symptoms:

- when they first occurred

- what they are like

- whether they are related to sexual intercourse

- whether you have had similar symptoms in the past

- whether you have any idea what you have.

You will also be asked if you have had any STD before, and if so what treatment was given. Some of the questions can be rather embarrassing, such as,

- how many sexual partners you have

- when you last had sex, and

- whether you have oral or anal intercourse.

Your answers will give the doctor valuable information on how you may have been infected, where, and whether there are other individuals who may also be infected, and therefore in need of treatment. The doctor, or a social health advisor will probably give you a contact slip to give to your partner(s) which they can then take to any clinic in the UK. The slip includes your clinic number and a code for the diagnosis. This will help the doctor who sees your partner decide on appropriate tests. If your contact is seen at a different clinic from you, the slip will be returned to the original clinic so that accurate contact tracing records can be kept.

Women are asked about their menstrual history and whether their symptoms appear to be related to their menstrual period. They will also be asked if they have had an abortion or miscarriage as these can be an indication of latent syphilis. All patients are asked about their contraceptive history and, specifically, whether or not a woman has an intra-uterine contraceptive device (IUD or coil) in place — since these increase the risk of pelvic inflammatory disease

After the interview you will be sent to an examination room, asked to undress from the waist down and to lie on the couch. A local genital examination is carried out, sometimes augmented by a general physical examination. Your external genitalia will be examined for evidence of disease; you will be asked to provide a blood and urine specimen (see Chapter 2) and the anus, urethra, and ureter may also be examined and specimens taken if necessary. Women will have a cervical smear (see Chapter 6), and specimens will be taken from the vagina and cervix. A bimanual examination (see Chapter 6) should also be performed.

Blood tests for syphilis are performed on all patients since this can be a concurrent asymptomatic infection. Laboratory tests on the specimens can be performed immediately at the clinic and a diagnosis obtained while you wait. Sometimes specimens have to be cultured and you will therefore be asked to return in three to seven days for the results. If a STD is diagnosed you will be given treatment at once. All treatment is free of prescription charges.

Before you leave the clinic you may be invited to talk with a social health worker to ask them any questions you may have. They will provide practical advice on avoiding STDs and preventing a recurrence. This interview is entirely optional.

CONCLUSION

With greater sexual freedom, more people are potentially at risk from sexually transmitted diseases. However, these conditions are easily diagnosed and many can be successfully treated. There are now many more places where sensitive, specialist help is available.

AIDS (ACQUIRED IMMUNE DEFICIENCY SYNDROME)

AIDS is one of the conditions that is caused by the Human Immunodeficiency Virus (HIV). HIV attacks the body's immune system making it vulnerable to infection and cancers that a healthy body would repel. These 'opportunistic infections' include rare forms of pneumonia (pneumocystis carinii pneumonia) and skin cancer (Kaposi's sarcoma). It is the infections, not AIDS that cause death.

Other conditions caused by HIV include:

- PGL (persistent generalized lymphadenopathy)

- ARC (AIDS related complex) various persistent symptoms, but no opportunistic infections. ARC is not necessarily fatal, although a significant proportion of those with ARC go on to develop AIDS.

- memory loss, personality disturbance and dementia — caused when HIV damages the brain rather than the immune system.

AIDS may be spread by

- sexual contact with an infected individual

- transfer of infected blood from one individual to another

- an infected mother to her newborn baby before or during birth or from breast milk

In Britain there are now over 1000 reported cases of AIDS and it is thought that there are as many as 40,000 people infected with HIV. 90% of AIDS cases in the UK are homosexual or bisexual men. The other 10% is made up of

- haemophiliacs and people who were infected by blood transfusions

- drug misusers who share infected needles

- **men and women who have had sex with an infected partner.**

It is these four groups who are most at risk from AIDS.

TESTING FOR AIDS

Unfortunately there is no test for AIDS. There is only the HIV antibody test. This is a blood test (see Chapter 2) which detects the presence or absence of antibodies to the virus. Whenever a new virus enters your blood stream, your blood builds up antibodies to fight it off. So a positive antibody test tells you that HIV has, at some point, been in your body and has caused the body to react to it. The test cannot determine whether you have AIDS or will develop AIDS in the future. It is assumed that anyone who is antibody positive can pass the virus on to others. All positive results are double checked.

A negative result should mean that no antibodies to HIV were found in the blood sample, but false negative results have been reported. It also takes your body about three months after infection to produce antibodies to HIV. So if you were tested shortly after having been infected — your test will be negative. A small number of people do not produce detectable antibodies to HIV and will therefore give a negative result to the test even if positive. A negative result is more reliable if you are not in any of the obvious at risk groups and have not had 'unsafe sex' or shared needles within the previous three months.

If you are worried that you might have the virus, you should think very carefully before taking the test. Will knowing you are HIV positive for example,

- **help your physical and mental health?**

- **make you more or less likely to infect others?**

For someone who is very anxious that they have been infected, having the test may be of benefit. Also knowing you are HIV positive does give you a chance to alter your lifestyle in ways that might reduce your chances of developing AIDS. For example, women in high-risk groups who are thinking about becoming pregnant or are in the early stages of pregnancy may benefit from having the test because of the risks to themselves (increased chances of developing AIDS) and to the child (contracting HIV) if they are HIV positive.

However, there are many people who feel there is little point in taking the test because

- there is no effective treatment available for those who are HIV positive

- the advice offered is the same whether the test is positive or negative

- the devastating effects a positive result will have on your life, regardless of whether or not you will go on to get AIDS

Once the test is done, you may lose control of what happens to the result. You should decide before taking the test whether the benefits are worth the risks. You should also discuss confidentiality with the person performing the test.

At an STD clinic, the results should remain confidential, although the clinic will want to tell your GP if the results are positive. Problems result if you are sent to another department within the same hospital; the specialist there will probably be told your result. This is then likely to go into your general hospital notes which are less confidential than those of STD clinics.

If your GP has your result, it is at his/her discretion whether or not it remains secret within the practice — for example by keeping the result apart from your general medical notes. As with STD clinics the GP must have your written permission to give the result to anyone else. Find out if your result will be mentioned in any reports to employers or insurance companies. At present, no major insurance company will accept anyone who is antibody positive for any type of life insurance.

Advice and counselling before and after having an HIV antibody test is now available from a variety of organizations, including the Terrence Higgins Trust (01 833 2971), the Haemophilia Society (01 407 1010), and by telephone from the London Lesbian and Gay Switchboard (01 837 7324).

Should you decide to have the test there are a number of places you can go

- any STD clinic

- your own GP

- people with haemophilia, and their partners, can arrange for the test through their Haemophilia Centre

- many private clinics offer confidential testing, costing around £50. Their accuracy of testing has not been assessed.

Wherever you go, expect to wait 3 to 8 weeks for the results.

The choice of having, or not having an HIV antibody test, may soon be denied us. A controversial decision was passed by a narrow majority at the annual representative meeting of the British Medical Association in July 1987. Doctors are now free to carry out HIV antibody tests on patients *without* their permission. Currently it may be criminal assault to take your blood for the HIV antibody test without your knowledge and consent. But this has yet to be tested in court. And by the time you find out that the test has been performed, the damage may already have been done.

Blood and semen donors are already screened for HIV, as are donors of kidneys, hearts, livers etc. With this new decision by the BMA, how close are we to the compulsory — perhaps secret — screening of people? AIDS has brought out the best and the worst in us. We see the courage with which sufferers struggle to come to terms with their condition, and we also see the ignorant bigoted way in which so many people react towards sufferers. Denying people such a basic freedom of choice is surely not the way in which a civilized society should react to what is in fact a rare condition that is difficult to catch. Let us hope that reason will prevail, and HIV antibody testing will continue to be used with the sensitivity and confidentiality it requires.

CONCLUSION

Testing for AIDS is in its infancy. We are still unsure of the significance of a positive result to the HIV antibody test. Is it really a death sentence? However, an enormous amount of research is being carried out all over the world, which should provide us with more informative diagnostic tests as well more successful methods of treatment.

UPPER AND LOWER RESPIRATORY TRACT CONDITIONS

As can be seen from the diagram, our respiratory system is divided into the upper and lower tract.

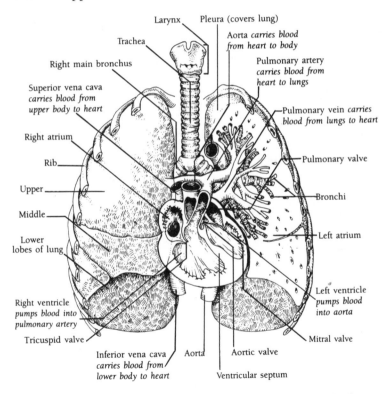

Larynx
Pleura (covers lung)
Trachea
Aorta *carries blood from heart to body*
Right main bronchus
Pulmonary artery *carries blood from heart to lungs*
Superior vena cava *carries blood from upper body to heart*
Pulmonary vein *carries blood from lungs to heart*
Right atrium
Rib
Pulmonary valve
Upper
Middle
Bronchi
Lower lobes of lung
Left atrium
Left ventricle *pumps blood into aorta*
Right ventricle *pumps blood into pulmonary artery*
Tricuspid valve
Mitral valve
Inferior vena cava *carries blood from lower body to heart*
Aorta
Aortic valve
Ventricular septum

Figure 15. The chest, showing the position of the lung and the heart.

Because of constant exposure to the outside environment, it is open to infection and inflammation; and we have all, at some

133

time, been affected, be it only a bout of flu. Respiratory diseases are extremely common, and include a wide range of conditions:

● infections and inflammations such as influenza, pneumonia, bronchitis, tonsillitis, tuberculosis, sinusitis, tracheitis, caused by bacteria or viruses

● allergic reactions such as asthma and hay fever

● cancer, particularly of the lungs

● emphysema

● blockages and clots, such as pulmonary embolism

When you go to your doctor with a suspected respiratory condition (s)he will be looking, among other things, for the following indications:

● cough

● shortness of breath

● chest pain

● swelling of the legs

Before any tests are ordered your doctor will perform a physical examination which will include:

palpation: careful feeling with hands and finger tips of the chest

percussion: tapping of the chest, with the fingers or an instrument to sense the resultant vibrations. This can, for example, detect the presence of fluid in the lungs

auscultation: listening, usually with the aid of a stethoscope to sounds produced by movements of gas or liquid within the body. It is useful, for example, in diagnosing abnormalities of the lungs according to the characteristic changes in sound pattern caused by different disease processes.

To confirm the diagnosis, the following tests may be ordered:

RADIOGRAPHY

Radiography has been immensely useful in the diagnosis of, and screening for, respiratory conditions and in screening for certain other conditions. A simple *chest X-ray* can provide enough information to confirm the doctor's diagnosis. Another commonly used radiographic technique is *bronchography*. Opaque iodised oil is introduced through a catheter into the lungs — via the trachea, under local or general anaesthetic. This highlights the bronchial tubes in subsequent X-rays — providing information about their size, location, and number. Bronchography is a fairly definitive test for bronchiectasis; but is also performed when certain other conditions are suspected, such as haemoptysis, lung sequestration and unilateral transradiancy.

Sometimes you will be asked to swallow a mixture containing barium ('Barium Swallow') in order to examine your throat and oesophagus. It is possible for the radiologist to use a fluoroscope (an instrument on which X-ray images may be viewed directly without taking and developing X-ray photographs) connected to a TV monitor to observe the progress of the barium through your body. Fluoroscopy is useful for the examination of heart, lungs and diaphragm in the dynamic state. It can help in the detection of blockages, abnormalities and tumours.

If your doctor wants to investigate suspected blood clots and other blockages of blood flow in the lungs (pulmonary embolism) he may order a *pulmonary arteriogram*. Contrast media is injected into your arm in order to outline the pulmonary arteries in the X-ray photographs.

CT SCANS

Despite considerable theoretical application to the lungs, little documentation is available on the value or accuracy of lung CT scans. Many doctors do feel that chest and lung diseases that were once very difficult to diagnose such as sarcoidosis, old hidden tuberculosis, enlarged arteries and veins can be detected by body scanning.

NUCLEAR SCANS

There are two types of scans which are used to investigate pulmonary function:

Perfusion scan detects blockages in the flow of blood from the heart to the lungs. The radioactive material is injected into your arm, and the scan monitors the blood flow.

Ventilation scan measures the flow of air in and out of the lungs. You are asked to inhale radioactive gas so that the scan can detect those areas of the lungs not receiving air. You will have to take a deep breath and hold it for approximately ten seconds to get a good image. This will be repeated over three to five minutes.

BRONCHOSCOPY

This technique allows the direct visualization of the bronchial tree under local, or general anaesthesia. The viewing instrument is inserted either through your mouth or nose. It is a useful tool in the diagnosis and investigation of lung cancer, and in the diagnosis of thoracic disease. Specimens for analysis can be taken at bronchoscopy. Performing a bronchoscopy can often reduce the necessity of more extensive exploratory surgery by allowing the doctor to directly view any abnormalities highlighted through X-rays or scans.

LARYNGOSCOPY

Laryngoscopy allows the doctor to investigate ear nose and throat problems. Most of the upper respiratory tract is visible. No anaesthetic is required unless the doctor needs a biopsy sample or is performing surgery. You may feel like gagging as the viewing instrument and mirror is placed in your throat, and the procedure is uncomfortable. It should not, however, be painful, so signal to your doctor to stop if it is. If a biopsy sample is taken, you may spit up a small amount of blood. If the bleeding continues, or you have breathing difficulties after the test, notify your doctor immediately.

LABORATORY ANALYSIS

Laboratory analysis of specimens taken from the infected area is one of the most important techniques in differentiating between respiratory conditions which all share similar signs and symptoms, and in the diagnosis of pulmonary disease. A variety of specimens may be taken for examination, analysis or culture.

Sputum is collected — when you cough it up, by bronchial washings or at bronchoscopy — if lower respiratory tract disease is suspected, there is a persistent cough that cannot be explained; or you have an undiagnosed general infection. Two other techniques for collection, not commonly used are

tracheal aspiration where a soft lubricated catheter is inserted through a nostril and down the throat to collect the specimen

transtracheal aspiration or tracheal tap in which the sample is collected through a needle inserted in the neck into the trachea

Throat swab is taken using a long cotton tipped swab, in order to test for throat infections.

Laryngeal swabs are also taken to test for infection and abnormalities

Pharyngeal or tonsillar swabs are often taken in order to diagnose common upper respiratory tract infections such as acute tracheitis and bronchitis

Tuberculin skin test This is a screening test to establish whether you have been infected by the bacteria that cause tuberculosis. A small amount of purified protein derivative from dead TB bacteria is injected into the skin on your arm, either by a doctor, nurse or trained technician. If you were infected with TB or vaccinated against TB in the past, your immune system will produce swelling at the injection site a day or two after the injection. The only risk with this test is an allergic reaction, should you ever have had contact with TB. There is no danger of contracting TB from the injection.

Pleural fluid To collect any fluid that may have accumulated in the space between the lungs and the pleura (a symptom of a number of respiratory disorders), a pleural tap will be performed. A needle is inserted through the chest wall, and fluid extracted, under local anaesthetic. As coughing may make the needle jerk and possibly injure your lungs, you may be given medication to suppress coughing prior to the test. An X-ray is sometimes performed after a pleural tap to ensure that the lung has not been punctured.

Blood tests Many tests can be performed on samples of your blood, in order to diagnose respiratory disorders. These are particularly useful in the diagnosis of TB, pneumonia, tonsillitus, emphysema, pulmonary embolism and various other viral infections.

URINALYSIS

The pH (measure of acidity of alkalinity) of your urine reflects the functioning of, among other things, your lungs. For example, lower than normal values may be a sign of emphysema.

BIOPSY PROCEDURES

(See Chapter 2 for details)
A biopsy may be necessary to confirm certain diagnoses — for example, of lung cancer. Various scoping procedures can be used to direct the biopsy (for example, thoracoscopy and mediastinoscopy), and depending on where the sample is being taken from, the procedure will be carried out under local or general anaesthetic. You should always discuss the risks and benefits of having a biopsy before agreeing to the procedure. The most commonly used biopsy techniques in the investigation of respiratory condition are *needle biopsy* under local anaesthetic (such as of the pleura, lungs, lymph nodes) and *open biopsy* under general anaesthetic (such as of the lungs and lymph nodes). Do ask your doctor if the least invasive technique could be used, if the biopsy is necessary.

PULMONARY FUNCTION STUDIES

Measurements of how well the lungs take in air, how much they can hold, how well they utilize air, and how well they can expel it are important in

- detecting and diagnosing lung disease

- evaluating abnormal lung function or abnormalities of the respiratory tract

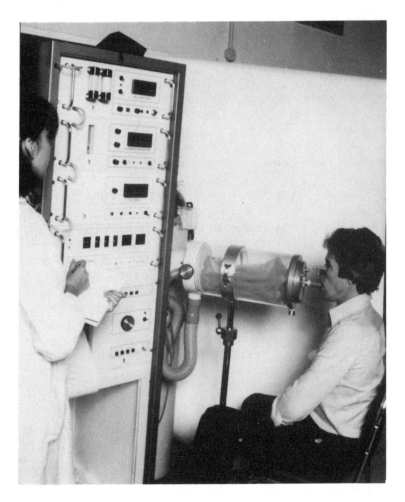

Figure 16. A man undergoing lung function tests.

- monitoring the progression of a known disorder

- determining how much of the lung can be removed in future surgery

Before undergoing these tests, there is some preparation. You will, for example, be asked to:

- avoid eating a full meal, for about four hours before the test, since a full abdomen restricts the movement of the diaphragm

- refrain from exercise and smoking for at least four hours before the test

- empty your bladder

- remove any dentures

- wear loose clothing

The tests should be explained to you beforehand, as the best results are obviously obtained if you understand what is required from you. If at any point during the tests you feel tired or faint, ask the doctor or technician performing them to stop. They will probably be performed in a specialist department within a hospital, although some of the simpler tests can be performed in a GP's surgery.

You will be asked to put on a nose clip to stop any air passing through your nose during the tests, and to place your lips tightly round the mouthpiece of the machine that measures the air you inhale and exhale. The exact instruction will vary according to the tests being performed.

The most common tests include:

forced vital capacity you will be asked to inhale as deeply as possible and then to blow all the air out as fast and hard as possible.

forced expiratory volume in one second is the amount of air you breathe out during the first second of a forced exhalation *maximum midexpiratory flow*   is the maximum rate at which air flows through your airways during a forced exhalation

maximum voluntary ventilation   this is the greatest amount of air you can breathe out during one minute.

Some tests may be repeated after you have inhaled a spray that helps expand your airways in the lungs. Or you may be given a carbon dioxide and air mixture to measure the ability of your lungs to exchange gases.

Pulmonary function tests are considered 90% accurate and are quite significant as there are very few false positive results. People in pain may not be able to breathe fully because of it, which may lead to misleading results.

ELECTROCARDIOGRAPHY

Certain heart conditions indicate certain pulmonary conditions, so an ECG may be performed (see Cardiology for details).

CONCLUSIONS

Respiratory conditions are common, but usually easy to diagnose. This means that where treatment is available it can be administered rapidly and with great effect.

Chapter 5

MAJOR AT RISK GROUPS

CHILDREN

It is in the area of children's medicine that the ethical problems regarding medical testing become most important and difficult. Clearly a medical test which involves some discomfort or pain, either emotional or physical, can create long-term psychological problems. Nevertheless, early diagnosis is particularly important with children as otherwise conditions left untreated may be potentially dangerous. The following factors must be borne in mind when considering performing a medical test:

- Is the test uncomfortable?

- Is the test cost effective?

- Is the test going to aid the diagnosis?

- Is the test without risk? If not is the risk worth the advantages?

- Apart from satisfying the desire for an accurate diagnosis is the test going to make a difference in treatment of the patient?

More and more medical tests are being performed, even on children, even though the only gain is the satisfaction of a correct diagnosis. Often, these tests make little or no difference to the management of the case and may even be potentially hazardous.

A typical example of this is an unnecessary X-ray. Children's bones do not break in the same way as adults' bones do, and frac-

143

tures are thus known as 'greenstick'. Minor greenstick fractures of the small bones of the hands and feet in children can often occur and present as pain, swelling and tenderness after an injury. These greenstick fractures readily heal and need no more than supportive bandaging, and thus an X-ray to confirm or deny whether a fracture is present makes no difference to the treatment of the patient. Nevertheless, possibly in view of the potential aspect of litigation, X-rays for such fractures are almost invariably performed despite the known hazards of X-ray examination, particularly in the young.

Obviously a painless, risk-free and cost-effective test which prevents any future problems is worth while. For example, at no age is screening more important although it is the middle aged who seem to consider that in some way screening can be a preventative measure. There are a number of conditions in childhood which, if detected in the first few weeks of life or immediately after birth, can dramatically alter the outlook for that patient. Because of this there are normal examinations and tests carried out throughout childhood, with other examinations and tests being performed if indicated.

There are three basic causes of conditions which are found in childhood: these are HEREDITARY conditions, CONGENITAL conditions and ACQUIRED conditions.

Hereditary diseases are those which are inherited from one or both parents. Some of these are actually present in the parent or parents, but more often occur when both parents, though themselves healthy, are carriers of the disease. In families where there is a particularly high incidence of a congenital condition it is now possible to identify carriers. Examples of hereditary diseases are cystic fibrosis and phenylketonuria (see below). Some diseases, whilst not directly hereditary in that a gene carrying the condition has been identified, seem to 'run in families' (for example, diabetes).

Congenital diseases are conditions which are not hereditary, but are present from birth. Abnormal heart structure and dislocation of the hip are examples — prediction of the condition is not possible from family history or examination of the parents.

Acquired diseases are those which appear after birth and are irrespective of hereditary factors. Common infections are obviously acquired, though there may be an underlying congenital or hereditary condition which aggravates them.

Tests on the newborn are designed to detect congenital or hereditary conditions, whereas those performed later in life look for acquired disease.

TESTS ON NEW BORN CHILDREN

Tests performed on new born and young children are designed to pick up any congenital abnormality or any congenital inborn error of metabolism. The former are the structural defects which occur, and may be major or minor, from a defective heart to a skin blemish. The inborn errors of metabolism are a group of conditions, genetically caused, which lead to various growth defects, either mental or physical, and which when detected are fully amenable to treatment

Immediately after birth all children in the UK are examined by a doctor to ascertain whether there are any congenital defects present. He or she will examine the digits, hands (children with Down's syndrome often show abnormal palmar creases) the limbs, the back (to detect for spina bifida) skull, eyes, mouth (for skin blemishes), and the hips and heart.

CONGENITAL DISLOCATION OF THE HIP

This condition arises where during development, the top end of the thigh bone is imperfectly placed in the socket of the pelvis, and if not detected early in life, leads to a permanent limp and stiffness of the hip. Early examination of the hips can detect this, and treatment with plaster splinting can set the joint in the correct fashion.

Other tests are only carried out in the new born if indicated (for example, by the family history) but one blood test is routinely performed. Approximately a week after birth a blood test is taken to detect phenylketonuria (PKU).

PHENYLKETONURIA TEST

Phenylketonuria is an enzyme deficiency which is inherited, in which the body is unable to metabolize an amino acid known as phenylalanine. Phenylalanine is a common constituent in proteins in the diet. If phenylalanine builds up in the blood stream, mental retardation can develop. PKU occurs approximately once in every 10,000 births and is most common amongst people from Northern Ireland and Scotland. A simple blood test (the Guthrie test) shows a raised level of phenylalanine and if the diagnosis is confirmed a diet low in phenylalanine will prevent the development of the mental retardation. Clearly as this test is easy (a heel prick is used to extract a drop of blood), relatively cheap, almost without discomfort and risk, and yet can prevent considerable handicap in later life, it is an example of a worthwhile test.

DEVELOPMENTAL CHECKS IN THE FIRST FIVE YEARS OF LIFE

In this country checks on infants are normally carried out by health visitors at 11 days, monthly until nine months, and then every six months. A full check is carried out at three years and four and a half years. Normally the health visitor will perform these and refer if necessary. These checks are mainly concerned with the growth rate but also with intellectual development, speech development, hearing and visual ability. They are the best form of screening examinations, in that they are devoid of risk or discomfort and yet can discover early problems requiring treatment.

NORMAL GROWTH DEVELOPMENT

A child's growth rate depends on many factors, and it is therefore impossible to state what an average for a child of a particular age would be. Charts of height and weight (see figures 17A, B, C and D) can give a guide to the development of a child over a period of time, but should be used in conjunction with other factors. On these charts the line marked 50 indicates the average growth in height and weight. However lines marked three and 97 indicate the levels at which only 3% will be below the lower line and only 3% will be above the upper line. Serial estimations

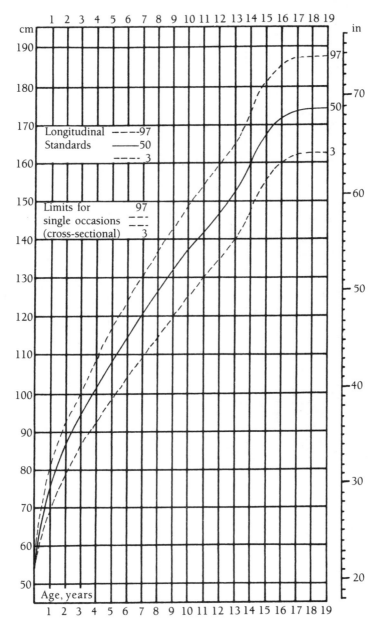

A Boys' Height

Figure 17. Charts showing children's average height and weight.

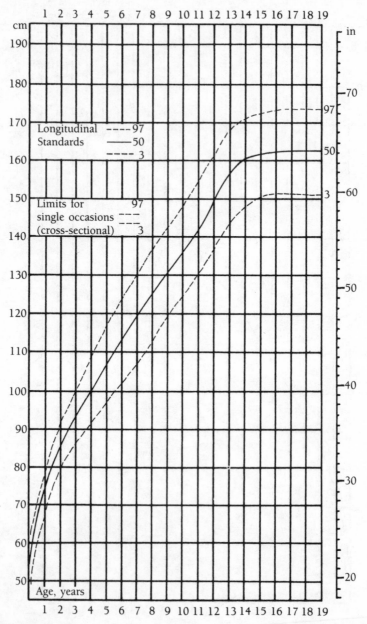

B   Girls' Height

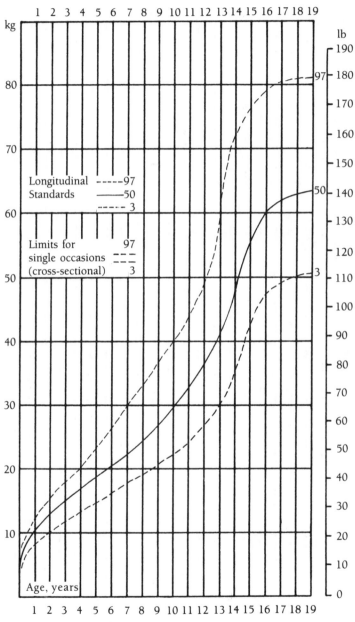

C   Boys' Weight

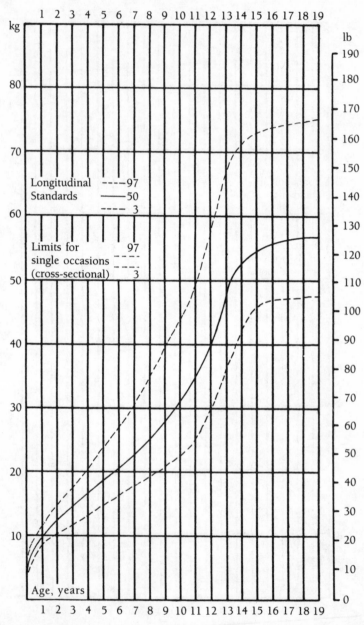

D Girls' Weight

using these charts are essential as a change from one area to another is of greater significance than a continuation of a line which may not be within the 'normal range'.

For this reason other charts which indicate the normal speed of growth are used. These show the rate of change of weight or height in kilograms or centimetres per year. A deterioration in a child's growth rate is of greater significance than his weight or height at a particular time, and a sudden alteration in growth rate may indicate a serious problem developing.

POOR WEIGHT GAIN IN INFANCY

If an infant in the first year of life fails to maintain a growth rate of at least 75% of that expected, further investigations are indicated. However the causes for failure to gain weight in infancy are numerous:

Underfeeding Although poor infant feeding is mainly prevalent in other parts of the world it still exists in the UK despite the Welfare State. Such a cause should be obvious from a careful assessment of the infant's diet.

Chronic infection in infancy This may be a cause of failure to thrive, or it may be a secondary effect due to the poor defence mechanism of the body as a result of the infection.

Congenital abnormalities of structure Abnormal structural development of organs (for example, a heart defect) which may not have been detected at birth can give rise to failure to maintain a normal growth rate. Examinations elsewhere for adults (for example, ECG and X-ray examination) can be carried out is such cases.

Pyloric stenosis This occurs where the exit from the stomach is narrowed, causing restriction of the outflow leading to malabsorption of food and persistent vomiting. Failure to survive results.

Cystic fibrosis This condition causes interference with nutrition by deficient intestinal absorption owing to poor release of enzymes from the pancreas. It is also associated with thick mucus in the lungs leading to lung infections. It is an inherited condition, but both parents may be healthy, and unaware that they are carriers of the disease. Cystic fibrosis can be diagnosed by means of the sweat test, which shows up the excessive amount of sodium in the sweat present in cystic fibrosis. However there are newer tests which can detect cystic fibrosis during pregnancy via amniocentesis (see page 175) in which enzymes can be detected.

Metabolic disorders There are a wide variety of genetically caused metabolic disturbances which are relatively rare and which may cause failure to thrive in infancy. These are discussed in Chapter 4 under metabolic and endocrine disorders. One common metabolic disorder is coeliac disease which presents with persistent diarrhoea and failure to thrive in the first year of life. It is due to an intolerance to gluten, a constituent of most cereals, and can be detected by biopsy of the small intestine. In this test, a small capsule at the end of a tube is passed into the stomach and subsequently into the intestines. A small hole in the side of the capsule allows part of the lining of the small intestine to be sucked into the capsule and removed with a built in knife. This can then be extracted and examined under the microscope.

Food intolerance Although this is still a contentious subject, most doctors now accept that cow's milk intolerance, leading to poor growth and intestinal disturbances, is a genuine complaint. It may be that in the future other foods will be recognized as causing intolerance.

VISUAL AND HEARING TESTS

Clearly tests for vision and hearing usually demand, for their accuracy, co-operation of the patient and an ability to express himself/herself. Therefore hearing and visual tests in very young children are limited to the detection of severe abnormalities.

HEARING TESTS

In the first year of life the health visitor will normally screen for a marked hearing loss by shaking a rattle behind the baby at one of the examinations (usually at nine months) and discovering whether the baby turns to the source of the sound. This test is sufficient to detect severe deafness (as may occur in congenital rubella).

AUDIOMETRY

Older children can have their hearing acuity tested by the audiometer. This is a machine which produces pure tones on different frequencies and allows the volume to be slowly increased until the child indicates that he/she can hear it. The pure tones vary from approximately 60 cycles per second (which correspond to low bass tones) to approximately 10,000 or 12,000 cycles per second which are very shrill or high whistles. The human ear can hear from 60 to 16 thousand cycles per second, although in childhood this may be increased to as much as 20 thousand per second.

The intensity of any sound is expressed in decibels. A whisper is approximately 20 decibels, loud classical music is produced at about 80 decibels and a jet engine may be over 140 decibels. Any continuous sound in excess of 85 decibels can cause temporary hearing loss, but if the human ear is subjected to this volume for any length of time, a permanent hearing loss could result.

For the test the child wears a pair of headphones, and each tone is slowly increased in volume until he/she indicates that he can hear it. The different levels (or decibels) at which he can hear the tone are then recorded on a specially prepared chart, which also indicates the normal range. This is approximately two decibels at 60 cycles per second and 10 decibels at 12,000 cycles per second.

There are many different kinds of hearing loss: some people only show the inability to hear high tones and some only low tones. Following excessive noise exposure, high tones are usually lost, whereas when deafness is inherited, hearing for the entire range is missing.

The ability to hear depends on two mechanisms. Normally sound is heard via air transmission, that is the waves travelling through the air cause movements on the eardrum which are transmitted to the inner ear and detected by the nerve to the ear. However, sound can also be detected if it is applied directly to the bone, causing the bone to vibrate, transmitting the sound

153

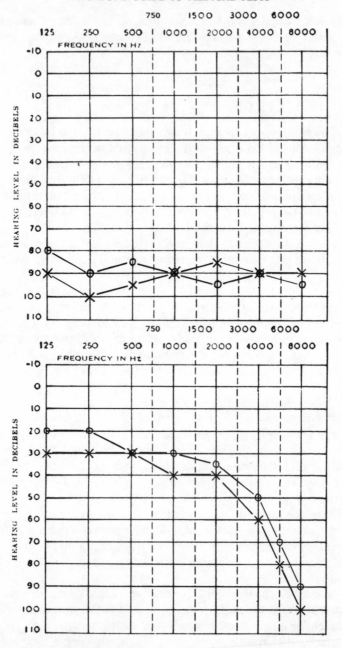

Figure 18. Audiograms showing severe hearing impairment (top) and high tone loss (bottom).

directly to the hearing mechanism, avoiding the external ear. In a normal patient the bone conduction is more acute than the air conduction, and a tuning fork applied to the bones of the skull, particularly behind the ear, will take the sound direct to the inner ear bypassing the middle and external ear.

Occasionally it is useful to estimate whether it is bone or air conduction which is lost. A patient who has lost the ability to hear by bone conduction is suffering from nerve deafness, whereas a person who retains bone conduction but is unable to hear by air conduction has a problem with the middle or external ear.

A more recent form of audiometry is now available, and this can be used in much younger children, even the new born. This is called evoked response audiometry (ERA).

This test uses an electro-encephalogram as a means of detecting the ability of the patient to hear sounds. An even more refined version of this is now available where needles are inserted into the part of the ear which 'hears' directly and a recording can be made of its activity when sound is passed into the ear.

VISUAL TESTS

Severe visual problems are normally obvious to the parents, but usually some underlying cause is apparent in the appearance of the eyes.

STRABISMUS (SQUINT)

In the first year of life a baby may appear to have a squint, in that one eye is turned inwards. This can be a mistake on the part of the parents, as many babies have marked epicanthic folds (folds of skin between the nose and eye which cover up the inner part of the eye and give the appearance of a squint). An easy test to discover the presence of a squint is to cover each eye in turn while the baby's gaze is fixed on some object. If a squint exists then when the normal eye is covered, the inturning eye will move to look at the object. This develops when one eye is markedly dominant over the other and the non-dominant eye loses the power of the muscles which control the eyeball.

TESTS FOR VISUAL ACUITY

Once a child is old enough to co-operate and express himself it is possible to accurately measure the degree of his visual acuity. The most common test uses the Snellen chart in which the patient reads a series of letters or numbers of various sizes from a distance of 20ft. For children unable to read or distinguish letters a circle with a gap facing one way can be used, like a large letter C facing forwards, backwards, up or down. A person with normal sight will see letters ⅜ of an inch high from a distance of 20ft. This visual acuity is recorded as 20/20. On the Snellen chart the largest letter is 3½ inches high, and if the patient can only read this letter at 20ft, the visual acuity is recorded at 20/200, indicating that someone with normal vision could read that letter 200ft away.

Defects in visual acuity usually fall into one of the following groups:

Myopia, or nearsightedness   Characterized by difficulty in seeing objects at a distance but ability to read or see objects close to. This occurs when the lens of the eye or the cornea are too curved.

Presbyopia, hyperopia or farsightedness   When people can see clearly at a distance but have difficulty reading close to. In these patients the lens is too flattened.

Astigmatism   When the eye cannot focus properly in certain lines across the field of vision, caused by a non-symmetrical shape to the cornea. These patients may therefore be able to see clearly all the numbers on a clock face except those at positions 1 and 7.

Anisometropia   This is a major difference in the visual acuity between the two eyes. In this condition one eye usually becomes dominant, and therefore strabismus (see above) can develop.

RETINOSCOPY

This is a much more objective way of testing vision and is therefore particularly suitable with children. A beam of light from an ophthalmoscope is focused on the back of the eye and lenses are placed in the beam to make the focus accurate. The strength of this lens is an indicator of the defect of the lens within the eye. There are now electronic devices which are based on this method that can detect visual problems within minutes.

More recently a new eye chart has been introduced that is more accurate than the standard Snellen chart. This uses circles and bars of different contrasts and can measure visual acuity under varying light conditions.

COLOUR BLINDNESS

The most common form of colour blindness is the inability to differentiate between red and green, and this affects approximately one in every 25 men (strangely the figure is one in every 250 women) and usually runs in families. A much more rare form of colour blindness is an inability to tell the difference between blue and yellow.

TEST FOR COLOUR BLINDNESS

This uses a series of coloured plates composed of dots of varying sizes and colours (usually known as Isahara plates). Most of them display a hidden letter or number within the dots, which is visible to a normal patient. People who are colour blind cannot distinguish certain plates. Hidden amongst the plates are usually two false plates in which normal people cannot usually distinguish a number. These are inserted in case patients are trying to fake a result.

FIELD OF VISION

A person of normal vision is clearly fully aware of objects and activities in the area immediately around him. This area is known as the field of vision, and extends for approximately 45 degrees each side and up and down when looking forwards. Certain conditions, especially undetected glaucoma, can affect this field of vision, and may be the first sign of a problem. Consequently an estimation of the field of vision is a common adjunct to visual acuity tests.

TESTS FOR FIELD OF VISION

There are two methods for testing the field of vision. In the older one, one eye is covered with a small plastic cup, and the eye is fixed on a mid point on a screen. The examiner then brings slowly in from the outside of this area a small disc on the end of a stick, and the patient states when it comes into his area of vision. This is a fairly time-consuming procedure, as it has to be repeated through all 360 degrees around the central point.

Even in the normal person there is a small area (known as the blind spot), within his field of vision, within which he can normally not see an object. This is due to the optic nerve and the point at which it becomes attached to the back of the eyeball.

A more modern test of field of vision involves a similar screen and fixation of the vision at the centre, but flashing lights are displayed in a particular sequence, and the patient states how many lights are visible. This is a much quicker though not necessarily more accurate method of assessment.

TESTS FOR THE COMMON DISEASES OF CHILDHOOD

WORMS

Parasitic infestation, particularly with thread worms, is relatively common in childhood. It frequently recurs and proves extremely difficult to eradicate.

Typically the child will complain of anal itching, especially at night. Frequently it is possible to see the worms at the anal entrance, looking like short white threads. A simple test for the presence of thread worms is the SCOTCH TAPE TEST in which a piece of adhesive tape is attached to a pencil with the sticky side out and run over the anus. This is then examined under a microscope and will display the presence of eggs if the worms are present.

The life cycle of the thread worm is such that recurrent infections are common. Children often scratch themselves at night, which results in the eggs being placed under the fingernails and then re-ingested via the food or through finger or thumb sucking during the day. Medication does not eradicate the eggs but only the adult worms and the condition can therefore persist.

MUMPS

Mumps is a viral infection (see below for general tests on viral infections) with an incubation period between 12 and 28 days. The symptoms are characteristically a swelling of the parotid glands, which develop enlargements at the angle of the jaw on both sides. Similar symptoms on other glands, particularly the pancreas and the testicles (in boys), can occur.

GLANDULAR FEVER

This condition (also known as mononucleosis) is relatively uncommon in childhood and more prevalent in teenagers. The symptoms are many and varied, and can include sore throat, headache, enlarged glands, abdominal pain, and occasionally neurological problems. As the clinical picture is not typical, blood tests are usually added to support the diagnosis. The main one consists in the detection of antibodies and an increase in abnormal lymphocytes in a blood cell differential (see Chapter 2).

MEASLES

This is another viral disease (see general test below) but testing is rarely necessary as the clinical picture is so typical. The incubation period is 10 to 14 days, and it commonly occurs at any age between eight months and five years. However in recent years introduction of measles vaccination has dramatically reduced its incidence.

GERMAN MEASLES

German measles or rubella is a viral infection with an incubation period of 14 to 19 days. It is a relatively mild illness causing lethargy, slight temperature rise and characteristic rash appearing on the face and spreading to the trunk and limbs. In addition, the glands around the neck and behind the ears are normally enlarged. As the condition is short and self limiting, sometimes its existence is missed. The significance of rubella are the complications which may develop if it is caught during pregnancy. Thus vaccination against rubella is advisable for girls and women who have not acquired immunity.

TONSILLITIS

Infection of the tonsils is usually caused by bacteria (normally a streptococcus), although it may be a viral illness. Diagnosis is confirmed by swabs being taken from the tonsils and cultured. Appropriate antibiotic therapy is indicated if a bacterial cause is shown.

CHICKEN POX

A mild viral illness for which testing is usually unnecessary as the rash is so typical. Small vesicles or blisters which are full of fluid appear on the skin and they subsequently burst and heal, usually with no scar. Smallpox when it was common (it has now been eradicated world-wide) produced similar but larger blisters.

VIRUS DISEASES IN CHILDREN

Viruses cause more disease than any other group of micro-organisms, and are a common cause of childhood illnesses. In the past it was often difficult to arrive at a specific diagnosis, and illnesses were frequently stated to be due to a virus without sufficient laboratory information. Now, however, there are many tests that can pinpoint the particular organism, or if not, can at least identify which family of viruses the suspect one belongs to.

TESTS FOR VIRAL DISEASES

The usual way to diagnose a specific virus caused condition is through a blood test. The serum is examined for specific antibodies to the suspected virus. However these tests rely on the estimation of the antibody which develops during the disease and remains elevated thereafter, hence a single estimation of a raised antibody level will only indicate that an infection has occurred at some previous time, not necessarily that this virus is now present. It is therefore usual for two different blood serum examinations to be performed at intervals of up to two or three weeks. If this is performed and a rising level of antibody is shown, then this is indicative of a recent or present infection with that virus. However sometimes an exceptionally high level of antibodies against a specific virus on a single blood test may be accepted as diagnostic. For a more precise diagnosis specific viruses can be cultured once they have been isolated from body specimens. Some of the virus groups and individual viruses and the diseases they cause are:

Adenovirus This causes nose, throat, lung, and gastointestinal diseases.

Arbovirus group These viruses cause encephalitis, eye and bladder diseases.

Chicken pox (varicella) The test for this virus helps differentiate among diseases producing rashes.

Coxsackie groups There are two distinct groups. Within group A there are 23 known types. Within group B, there are 6 known types. They cause lung disease, paralytic types of illness, and a heart disease in newborn infants that imitates congenital defects.

Cytomegalovirus Inflammation of pancreas and salivary glands.

Echovirus/Enterovirus Both belong to the same group and can cause poliomyelitis, meningitis, heart and lung conditions, diarrhoea and other gastrointestinal symptoms.

Hepatitis This causes inflammation of the liver.

Herpes Two types: one causes cold sores and genital herpes, whereas the second causes shingles.

Influenza and parainfluenza (flu) Influenza of the lungs is usually designated Type A, B or C; A and B are the most familiar. Type C is a very mild form of the 'flu'. Parainfluenza, a lung disease generally limited to very young children, is divided into Types 1, 2, 3, and 4.

Lymphocytic choriomeningitis Another form of meningitis.

Measles (rubeola) The test for this virus can distinguish between it and German measles (rubella) in pregnant women and newborn infants. The virus can, however, also cause encephalitis.

161

Mononucleosis (see p 159)

Mumps (parotitis) (see p 159). This virus causes infection and swelling of the salivary glands, as well as swelling and possible sterility of the testicles.

Reovirus At times, this is considered part of the echovirus group. The r stands for 'respiratory', the e for 'enteric' (gastrointestinal), and the o for 'organs'. This virus causes pneumonia and diarrhoea, especially in children.

Retrovirus A family of viruses associated with schizophrenia, and, more recently with AIDS.

Rotavirus The cause of gastroenteritis in children.

Syncytial The cause of pneumonia-like disease in young children.

INTELLECTUAL AND PSYCHO-LOGICAL TESTING IN CHILDREN

LEARNING DISORDERS

An inability to perform as well as other children may result from an inherited condition causing mental retardation, a physical handicap such as impaired hearing, vision or co-ordination, a developmental defect, or an allergy causing hyperactivity. There are numerous tests, previously mentioned, to detect such abnormalities, but there are some which are specifically designed to detect reduced learning ability or specific learning disorders such as dyslexia.

INTELLIGENCE TESTS

Most intelligence tests measure an individual's ability to learn as compared to that of the population at the same age, and is expressed as the IQ or intelligence quotient. This figure is aimed at by dividing the mental age as determined by the tests by the chronological age and multiplying the result by 100. Thus the average IQ at any age is 100. There are numerous IQ tests in use, some of which rely more on verbal ability and some on performance tests. It is now felt that a combined test of verbal and physical performance is a better assessment for overall IQ, as this allows for any deficiency in one area of learning to be made up by an improved ability in the other. In general, performance tests are considered to be best as predictors for adjustment, and verbal tests are better as predictors for educational achievement.

Generally speaking, IQs of between 90 and 100 are considered average. An IQ of over 140 is considered to be a genius level. IQs of less than 35 are considered indicative of severe mental retardation, between 35 and 50 of moderate mental retardation and of 52 to 67 of mild mental retardation.

TESTS FOR DYSLEXIA

Dyslexia is a difficulty in understanding the written word, and a tendency to mentally reverse printed letters and thus not comprehend the meaning of sentences. It is now the most common learning disorder, and its cause may lie in the brain or in the eyes. Specialized tests are now available in order to diagnose dyslexia, though their interpretation may at times be difficult and lead to an incorrect diagnosis.

OTHER LEARNING DISABILITIES

Writing disorders may result from a lack of co-ordination between the hand and the brain, which may not be related to dyslexia, and a problem with subjects involving memory (e.g. mathematics) may be due to a memory disorder rather than reduced intelligence or specific learning disabilities. Evaluation of these can only be made through proper testing.

CONCLUSION

In summary, tests in children should be directed at the identification of conditions which when diagnosed early can influence the quality or length of life, whether they are hereditary, congenital or acquired. They should not be used for clinical accuracy when this does not affect the outcome or the management.

PREGNANT WOMEN

PRECONCEPTUAL CARE

It is possible for prospective parents to improve their chances of producing an healthy child by concentrating on their own health prior to conception. The Foresight Association have suggested that prospective parents should have a comprehensive medical about six months before conception. This should include:

- For the mother:
  - a check for rubella immunity
  - gynaecological examination

- For both parents
  - blood sample to check for VD; abnormalities of thyroid function; transaminase activity as a test for pyridoxine deficiency, zinc concentration and blood lead levels. A blood film will be analysed to test for active allergic response
  - urine analysis to test for sugar and delat-aminolevulenic acid (indicitive of a high lead burden)
  - hair analysis to check levels of 21 metals
  - stools analysis for evidence of infestation or malabsorption

- For the father:
  - semen examination for presence of abnormal sperm.

PREGNANCY TESTS

Most pregnancy tests rely on the detection in the urine of the hormone human chorionic gonadotropin (HCG) which is produced when the fertilized egg attaches itself to the wall of the uterus. Pregnancy tests are most accurate when carried out two weeks after a missed period, but some lab tests can pick of traces of HCG a week to ten days after conception.

HOME TESTS

If the manufacturer's instructions are followed exactly home pregnancy tests can have a 95% accuracy rate. The instructions vary, but usually involve mixing two component parts with a specimen of your urine and noting changes in the resultant mixture. The result can be affected by a number of things, including certain drugs; the instructions should provide details of what to avoid. It is always advisable to have your result confirmed by a laboratory test. A negative test should be repeated one week later if there is any suspicion or fear of pregnancy.

LABORATORY TESTS

Laboratory pregnancy tests are performed free of charge by your GP, local hospital, or family planning clinic. Pregnancy advisory services sometimes charge as do family planning clinics if you are not a regular patient. Commercial laboratories also advertise pregnancy tests by mail order or while you wait. Their charges vary — and so can their accuracy. Some chemists will carry out the tests for a fee.

The result should be ready on the same day, but do check as hospitals and GPs can keep you waiting for a fortnight which is unacceptable.

You will be asked to provide either a sample of the urine you passed early in the morning or a blood sample. Blood tests can detect pregnancy as early as a week before the expected period is missed, but are more expensive so are only used if it is critical to recognize pregnancy at an early stage such as when an ectopic pregnancy is suspected.

OTHER PREGNANCY TESTS

Internal examination By means of a pelvic examination (see Chapter 6) your doctor can examine your cervix and uterus for evidence of pregnancy. The examination does not harm the embryo and is most commonly performed at the booking in clinic. From the eighth week a pelvic examination is extremely reliable in detecting pregnancy.

Ultrasound examination This can pick up pregnancy at six weeks and is particularly useful in detecting ectopic pregnancies.

Hormone pregnancy test A hormonal preparation (given by pill or injection) containing oestrogen can detect pregnancy before it can be confirmed by most conventional methods, by inducing withdrawal bleeding if you are not pregnant. However, you may bleed and still be pregnant and there is evidence that the test is harmful to the foetus. So if pregnancy is desired, this method should NOT be used.

Detecting an ectopic pregnancy Ectopic means that the foetus is implanted and growing outside the cavity of your uterus — most commonly in your fallopian tubes. The following tests are commonly used to diagnose ectopic pregnancies:

Culdocentesis (see Chapter 6)

Laparoscopy (see Chapter 6)

Human chorionic gonadotrophin test HCG will be present but the levels will not increase as they would with a normal pregnancy

Ultrasound blood counts and urinalysis may be taken to rule out other causes of the symptoms such as appendicitis, bladder infection and tumours.

ANTENATAL CARE

Once your pregnancy is confirmed your doctor will usually refer you to an antenatal clinic, either attached to a GP surgery/health centre or at your local hospital.

At your first visit (at around 12 weeks) you will be asked about your past medical and obstetric history to determine whether or not your pregnancy and delivery will be normal. A series of routine tests will then be performed.

Subsequent visits will be every four weeks until the 28th week, every two weeks to the end of the 36th week and from then onwards weekly until you go into labour.

ROUTINE TESTS

Test	Purpose	Significance
Height and shoe size (first visit)	Assessing size of pelvis and pelvic outlet	Small feet or height suggests a small pelvic outlet which may make delivery difficult
Weight (every visit)	Following foetal growth	Large weight loss will be investigated. Sudden weight gain may indicate pre-eclampsia
Breast (first visit unless there is a problem)	Checking for lumps and condition of the nipples	If nipples are retracted and you wish to breast feed you may be advised to wear a breast shield, or do gentle exercises
Heart, lungs, hair, eyes, teeth, nails, (first visit)	Checking on your general physical health	You may need some special attention and dietary supplements or just general advice on diet
Legs and hands (every visit)	1. Detection of varicose veins and any swelling (oedema) in the ankles, hands or fingers	Extreme puffiness can be a sign of pre-eclampsia

Test	Purpose	Significance
	2. Detection of blood clotting in the leg veins or pelvis	Thrombo-embolism is the second major cause of maternal death in Wales and England
Urine (Mid stream) (first visit)	Testing for kidney infection	An existing kidney infection you may not know you have can develop into a serious condition in pregnancy. You will be treated with antibiotics.
Urine (every visit)	1. Testing for protein	Protein in urine late in pregnancy is a sign of pre-eclampsia. Bed rest will probably be prescribed.
	2. Testing for presence of sugar	Pregnancy can unmask diabetes, which must be treated and stabilized. It may go away after delivery and only return in later pregnancies
	3. Testing for ketones	Presence of ketones indicates that the body is short of sugar, possibly due to diabetes
Internal exam (first visit)	1. To confirm the pregnancy and check the uterus is the size it should be according to the dates	Excludes problems with the cervix and the pelvic cavity

Test	Purpose	Significance
	2. To take a cervical smear	If cancer test is positive you will need to discuss the options with the obstetrician
	3. To check for pelvic abnormalities	Mention at the clinic if either you or your partner have ever suffered from genital herpes. If you have an active infection in the last week of pregnancy, you may be delivered by Caesarean section to avoid infecting the baby.
	4. To check that the cervix is tightly closed.	
Foetal heart rate (every visit)	To confirm foetal heart and heart rate are normal	
Abdominal palpations (every visit)	To assess the height of the fundus (the top of uterus) and the size and position of the foetus	Estimate the length of the pregnancy and the position of the foetus in the womb. If at 32 weeks the foetus has not turned from the breech position to the head first or cephalic position, the doctor may try to turn the baby by a process known as external cephalic version (ECV)

Test	Purpose	Significance
Blood pressure *(every visit)*	To assess if it is normal	Hypertension (high blood pressure) can indicate a number of problems including pre-eclampsia. Constant checks mean it can be kept under control if it suddenly rises eg above 140/90. May mean bed rest in hospital if it rises. Any rise in the lower or diastolic figure is cause for concern.
Blood tests *(first visit and once during third trimester)*	1. To find your major blood group ABO	Blood group needed in case of an emergency transfusion
		To check for blood group (ABO) incompatibility: when the mother is blood group O and her baby is A, B, or AB this may cause jaundice in the child
	2. To find your Rhesus blood group. Rhesus factor is a protein present in red blood corpuscles. 85% of Caucasians are Rh positive. The remaining 15% do not have the Rh factor; they are Rh negative	In case of Rhesus incompatibility where the baby is positive and the mother is negative

Test	Purpose	Significance
	3. To find your haemoglobin level (repeated test). This is a measure of the oxygen-carrying substances in your red blood cells. Normal levels, measured in gm, are between 12 and 14gm.	If your haemoglobin level goes below 10gm treatment for anaemia will be given. Iron and folic acid supplements will raise the level so that more oxygen can be carried to the baby
	4. To detect the presence of German measles antibodies	To find out whether or not you have immunity to rubella; if not you will be warned not to come in contact with German measles
	5. VDRL, Kahn or Wasserman tests for the presence of syphilis	If you unknowingly have had this sexually transmitted infection it is essential to treat it before week 20 of your pregnancy; after this time it can be passed to the baby
	6. To detect sickle cell disease and thalassaemia, both forms of anaemia found in dark-skinned people and inhabitants of Mediterranean countries	Can affect the baby and the pregnancy, hence the questions about race at the booking in, which may be offensive to some. Your blood will be tested for this disease if you are from a race which is affected by it. Extra folic acid will be

171

Test	Purpose	Significance
		prescribed and in extreme cases of sickle cell, a blood transfusion may be necessary

ANTENATAL SCREENING

Screening of all pregnant mothers, and high risk pregnancies, has had enormous impact on the prevention of birth disorders. In particular this has been true for Down's syndrome and foetal neural tube defects.

Before undertaking any antenatal screening of diagnostic procedure there are some very important issues that you and your partner should discuss with the obstetrician. Then, if you decide to go ahead, and the result arrives, you are better prepared to make the most appropriate decision. You should at least consider the following:

Foetal disorder:

- its severity

- long-term problems for the child, yourself and the community if an affected infant survives

- the possibilities and effectiveness of treatment

- the possibilities of the occurrence or recurrence of the disorder

Risks:

- of the technique to mother and foetus:

- the chances of misdiagnosis or failed diagnosis

Procedures:

- what it involves

- the time interval before a diagnosis can be made

Options:

- advantages and disadvantages of having the test

- if you have the test and it is positive, what you can do

- what should you do about future pregnancies

ANTENATAL SCREENING AND DIAGNOSTIC TECHNIQUES

ULTRASOUND

Ultrasound produces a very accurate picture of the foetus in utero. The first scan is done at about 12 to 14 weeks and then at any time during pregnancy after that. Some centres do not have this equipment but you will be referred elsewhere for a scan should medical staff think that it is necessary. For details see Chapter 2.

- **Ultrasound is used to:**

    - measure the age and growth of the baby to determine the estimated date of delivery

    - find the exact position of the baby and placenta prior to amniocentesis

    - locate the position of the placenta and its condition, should it become dislodged late in pregnancy

    - determine if you are carrying more than one baby (usually carried out in the first trimester). An X-ray is sometimes necessary in the 32nd to 34th week to check the relative positions of the babies, their relative sizes and abnormalities, if any.

    - pick up visible abnormalities of the baby such as brain and kidney conditions

- identify any growths in the mother that might hinder delivery
- diagnose an ectopic pregnancy
- diagnose foetal heart defects

Most doctors believe that ultrasound is safe, and that it does not affect the foetus. However, there is some evidence that there is a higher incidence of dyslexia and learning disorders in children whose mothers were given ultrasound during pregnancy. The US National Institutes of Health Consensus Panel, after reviewing the use of ultrasound in pregnancy, recommended that it should not be used as a routine test as it was unclear that, if used as a general test it did improve perinatal outcome or decrease morbidity and mortality. The World Health Organization have concluded that the use of ultrasound in pregnancy appears to have been introduced on a wide scale without appropriate evaluation of its benefits, safety or costs.

FOETOSCOPY

This is a recent addition to high technology obstetrics. It should not be used unless absolutely necessary, as it carries with it significant risks: one in eight women who undergo foetoscopy will lose a normal baby. See Chapter 2 for details of scoping procedures.

Foetoscopy is usually carried out in week 15 of the pregnancy and is used to check for brain abnormalities, blood disorders and any visible defects such as cleft palate. Your doctor should explain the risks to you before you give your consent to this test.

AFP SCREENING

Alpha feto protein is found in the blood of a pregnant woman in varying levels throughout the pregnancy. The levels should be low between weeks 16 and 18; any rise found at this time may indicate that you are carrying a baby with a neural tube defect such as spina bifida or other abnormalities of brain development. However, this is not a definitive diagnostic test and to be sure of a defect, alpha feto protein must be found in the amniotic fluid through an amniocentesis. Sensitivity in detecting spina bifida is only about 80% which is distressing to those women who have a normal test result but still give birth to a spina bifida child.

AFP may also rise with a twin pregnancy, threatened pregnancy, or where the foetus is not growing properly. It also rises naturally as the pregnancy progresses, so the doctor may check using ultrasound to see if your levels are high because the pregnancy is more advanced than originally thought.

AMNIOCENTESIS

Amniotic fluid contains cells from the skin and other organs of the foetus which can be analysed for a wide variety of genetic disorder, including:

- Down's syndrome

- spina bifida

- anencephaly

- factor Viii and factor 1 haemophilias

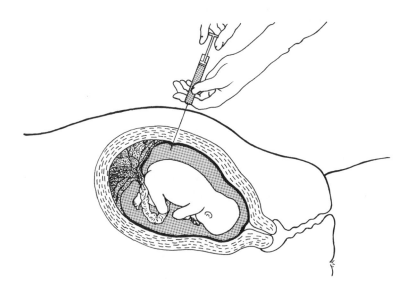

Figure 19. Diagram to show the extraction of a sample of amniotic fluid.

- Duchenne muscular dystrophy

- common haemoglobinopathies: sickle cell disorders and thalassemias

Amniocentesis is performed if:

- the mother is over 35, because of the increased risk of chromosomal abnormalities, especially Down's syndrome

- the couple already have an abnormal child

- a Caesarean section is planned: Tests will reveal the maturity of the baby's lungs. Immature lungs may be affected by respiratory distress syndrome

- raised AFP levels have suggested spina bifida

- there is a case of rheus incompatibility

- there is a history of previous miscarriages

Amniocentesis should not be performed simply to establish the sex of a child.

Amniocentesis is usually carried out 14 weeks after the last menstrual period in order to ensure that there is sufficient fluid in the amniotic sac, and therefore cells to analyse. It is performed as an out-patient procedure.

You will have been asked to empty your bladder before the procedure. An ultrasound scan should be used to determine the position of the foetus and the placenta as this reduces the chance that the doctor will fail to obtain amniotic fluid. Then a small area of the abdomen is treated with local anaesthetic and a long hollow needle is inserted into the womb. About 14g of fluid is withdrawn from the amniotic sac and sent to the laboratory for examination. The foetal heart beat should be ascertained both before and after the procedure. Since the maternal bladder is occasionally penetrated instead of the amniotic sac, the aspirated fluid is usually checked before the amniocentesis needle is withdrawn.

The cells are cultured for two and a half to five weeks. There is also a chance (between 4-10%) that the cultures will fail — usually because there was too much foetal blood present, and you will be asked to return for a repeat test. You therefore have to be prepared for quite a long wait before your results are ready.

It is difficult to assess the risk of miscarriage as a result of amniocentesis, but a realistic figure is probably about 4%. It has been suggested that amniocentesis should not be offered to women who have clinical signs of threatened abortion to give the foetus a better chance of survival. There is also a slight risk of infection — indicated by abdominal pain, chills, fever or leakage of fluid or blood from the vagina or puncture site.

The decision to have amniocentesis should be weighed up against the reasons for you being offered it at all and whether you are prepared to have your pregnancy terminated if the results give cause for concern.

If you are having an amniocentesis check what tests will be done on the withdrawn fluid — sometimes it will be tested for only one abnormality and may not pick up other problems that might be there. Insist on any tests that could apply to you.

CHORIONIC VILLI SAMPLING/BIOPSY

This is a new technique which is currently being evaluated in this country — with a sample of 4000 women. Depending on the results it may replace amniocentesis as a method of screening for genetic disease. The advantages are that the test can be performed at eight to eleven weeks and provide results within a few days. However, it may be that there is a higher risk of miscarriage and the accuracy of CVS needs to be compared with amniocentesis.

CVS involves the insertion of a thin hollow tube through the vagina and cervix into the uterus. Small tissue samples are taken by suction of the chorion, a layer of tissue surrounding the amniotic sac and the foetus. This tissue contains cells which have a genetic composition similar to that of the foetus.

FOETAL BLOOD SAMPLING

Samples of foetal blood obtained in utero can be used for the prenatal diagnosis of a number of conditions. A needle, guided using ultrasound, is used to obtain the sample.

FOETAL TISSUE SAMPLING

Foetal skin and liver have been sampled successfully and used for histologic and biochemical studies when amniocentesis or foetal blood sampling could not provide the necessary information. Biopsy instruments have been introduced under both fetoscopic and ultrasound guidance to collect these samples. Genetic skin disorders have been diagnosed in skin specimens. Certain metabolic disorders and deficiencies can be diagnosed with liver tissue.

PLACENTAL FUNCTION TESTS

These tests are performed on samples of your urine and blood to check the efficiency of the placenta, and can also monitor the baby's development and detect certain abnormalities.

DAILY FOETAL MOVEMENT COUNT

Daily foetal movement count is used as an alarm signal for foetal stress. The mother counts the number of times the foetus moves. Once she has counted ten she can stop as the child is normal;

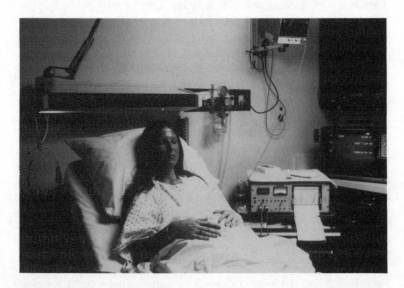

Figure 20. The equipment used for foetal monitoring during pregnancy and labour.

less than four a day should be reported to your doctor. Babies are most active between the 29th and 38th weeks, after which they quieten down. Self monitoring of foetal movements is usually carried out in the last 12 weeks of pregnancy.

ELECTRONIC FOETAL MONITORING (EFM), NON-STRESS TEST

This may be used to assess foetal well-being during pregnancy — usually from the 35th week. A transducer is moved along the mother's abdomen; when the foetal heart is located, the baby's pulse is heard on the amplifier. When the baby is very active the transducer has to be moved continually to keep up with it. Alternatively an external monitoring belt can be applied. The results show how your baby responds to its own movements.

EFM is useful for mothers whose pregnancies are at risk:

- older mothers carrying a first child

- pregnancies after long period of infertility

- mother with high blood pressure or diabetes

- when the child has stopped growing in the womb.

About one in seven such high risk pregnancies will show an abnormal EFM, less than 1 in 400 normal pregnancies will show an abnormal EFM, so it is not a cost effective routine test.

For EFM to be effective it must be used frequently as the EFM tracing can be normal one moment and abnormal the next.

EFM — STRESS TEST (OXYTOCIN CHALLENGE TEST)

Two external monitoring belts are applied to measure your baby's heart rate. You are given a small dose of the drug oxytocin through an intravenous (IV) needle to make your uterus contract. The baby's response to uterine contractions is then observed in order to see whether, when you actually give birth, everything will be normal. On very rare occasions this test may result in premature labour.

VALUE OF ANTENATAL CARE

Few studies have assessed the value of antenatal care — it has just been assumed to be a 'good thing'. Studies so far conducted have this to say:

● lack of antenatal care does not seem to have any detrimental consequence

● antenatal care is often ineffectual in identifying women at risk of complications in pregnancy and/or labour

● antenatal care has failed in its role of education — most women voicing dissatisfaction in their doctors ability to answer questions or indeed listen to them in the first place, thus increasing, rather than allaying anxiety and fear particularly in large hospital based clinics

● antenatal care has failed to attract women from classes other than the educated middle class

TESTING DURING LABOUR

The amount of testing will depend on where you have your birth and whether you fall into a high-risk category.

Periodic internal examinations are carried out during all labour to check that the right changes are occurring to the cervix, and that it is dilating at an appropriate rate. This is usually done with you lying flat on your back, but if this is uncomfortable ask if it can be done with you lying on your side.

FOETAL MONITORING

Various techniques have been developed to monitor the foetus during labour in order to detect foetal distress early enough for the baby to be delivered before coming to harm. These include:

- examination of the liquid observed following the rupture of the membranes or through the amnioscope. Foetal well-being can be assessed from the content of the liquid, but this is not a particularly accurate test.

- monitoring foetal heart rate. Changes in foetal heart beat are a good indication of some sort of foetal distress, so monitoring the foetus during labour should, so the argument goes, provide the doctor with an early warning system that will allow early diagnosis and treatment of intrapartum asphyxia with its attendant risks of still birth, neonatal death, or long-term handicap.

There is deep controversy about many aspects of foetal monitoring, in particular the introduction of electronic foetal monitoring as a routine procedure in labour.

Traditionally, the foetal heart beat was measured with a stethoscope for one minute in every fifteen. However, only 15% of foetuses in whom the diagnosis of distress was made with a stethoscope have biochemical evidence of asphyxia. This method is also not very sensitive — only an average heart rate can be counted, and it is difficult to listen to the heart at the most critical times — during contractions.

Today electronic foetal monitoring (EFM) can be used to record foetal heart beat — and the contractions of your uterus. It allows continuous, and more sensitive monitoring of beat to beat variations.

EXTERNAL ELECTRONIC FOETAL MONITORING

Electrodes are attached to your chest, two straps are also placed around your abdomen. The upper belt holds the tocodynameter, which records the intensity of the uterine contractions, and the lower strap holds an ultrasonic transducer, which monitors and records the foetal heart rate. This technique is between 90 and 95% accurate. When the ultrasonic device is not used, the external monitor is only about 57% accurate.

The straps can be uncomfortable and even painful, and can make it difficult to change position, and abdominal massage — which can be so helpful during contractions — becomes impossible. In any event, being strapped down is not conducive to producing the most efficient contractions.

INTERNAL ELECTRONIC FOETAL MONITORING

This is thought to be about 90% accurate. The technique relies on electrodes connected to wires within a plastic tube, which are introduced into your vagina and usually attached directly to the baby's head, by means of metal clips or screws. No studies have been done to establish whether this causes pain to the baby. These electrodes measure the baby's heartbeat. Your contractions are measured either by a catheter, introduced into your uterus through your vagina, or by the external strap described above.

Risk of infection and complications are greatly increased using this method, particularly if a uterine catheter is being used since to apply the internal electrodes your amniotic sac must first be ruptured. The baby can be at risk too — from bleeding due to the way the screw or clip is attached.

Both techniques require the monitoring of your blood pressure — measured by means of a blood pressure cuff attached to one of your arms. An intravenous solution and/or an induction drip are commonly attached to the other arm. Consequently your movements are severely restricted. Despite this some women do find the constant monitoring reassuring.

EFM has received an enthusiastic welcome from the medical profession — so much so that in some quarters, particularly the US, it is recommended for use in all labours. There are others though, who question its value and point out that little is known of its side effects. It is unclear what advantages there are to EFM in low risk pregnancies.

It would be interesting to know how much foetal distress is a result of the routine use of high technology machinery and unnatural procedures, rather than an intrinsic problem.

EFM certainly has a role in some circumstances, for example:

- when the labour is induced or accelerated

- if an epidural is used

- if you are diabetic or have high blood pressure

- the labour is premature

You should however, discuss its appropriateness to your own situation before agreeing to its use in your labour.

Disadvantages of EFM include:

- the staff are more aware of any small changes and therefore are more likely to intervene

- three times as many babies who are electronically monitored are delivered by Caesarean section

- EFM greatly increases the electronic paraphernalia in the delivery room

- staff are concentrating on the machine more than on the woman in labour

- EFM restricts movements thus slowing down the labour and making foetal distress more likely

- it may hurt the baby's head when the electrode is attached.

TELEMETRY

This measures radio waves. This technique allows the mother to walk about remote from the monitoring equipment. The electrode is still attached to the baby's head but it is joined to the mother's thigh and not to a large machine. However, babies do suffer rashes where the electrode was clipped to them and there is no proof that they feel no pain.

POST-NATAL CARE

Once the baby is born it will be given a thorough medical examination by a paediatrician. You should be informed of the results. Your temperature will be checked regularly to make sure you are not developing a puerperal (pertaining to childbirth) infection.

Your pulse will also be checked and you will be given a blood test after a day or so.

A midwife has to attend you by law for the first ten days after the birth. About 14 days after the birth a health visitor will take over from her. They will be able to monitor your health during this period.

Six weeks after the birth you should have a postnatal check up. You will be asked

- how you are coping

- if you are feeling miserable or depressed

- if you are suffering any discomfort or pain

- if your blood loss is still continuing

- if you are managing feeding

- if the baby is thriving

Both you and your baby should be given a thorough medical examination including urine, weight, blood pressure, blood tests. An internal examination should be made to check the uterus is returning to its normal size and a cervical smear may be taken. Any pain or discomfort should be dealt with. Your breasts should be examined to make sure that all is going well, whether you are breast feeding or not. Contraception should be discussed at this visit, if you do not wish to become pregnant immediately.

CONCLUSION

The medical profession have yet to find a balance between viewing pregnancy and birth as normal events not medical conditions, and providing help to those for whom the normal event is a risk, or where problems have occurred. There are now a number of screening and diagnostic techniques which are of great value to 'at risk' mothers, but which are often used unnecessarily on women whose pregnancies and births are without complications. Until such a balance is achieved, it is up to each woman to question the use of every technique and test they are asked to undergo before agreeing to its implementation.

ELDERLY PEOPLE

THE RELEVANCE OF TESTING

What are the medical profession to do? While ageing is a process not a disease, it does bring with it many medical problems. How much testing should be done on a sick old person? Medical investigation can find conditions which are treatable, making the old more able to live full and independent lives. So age alone should never be a sole criterion for determining the appropriateness of any test. A doctor must strike a balance between his/her desire for certainty and the value of the diagnosis to the elderly person: ie can anything be done for the person if the test is positive?

In early life the symptoms and signs of illness can usually be explained by a single diagnosis, but in old age diagnosis is compromised by the presence of more than one disorder. It has been said that if clinical examination of a sick old person does not reveal at least three or four pathological conditions, the patient has not been properly examined!

Many disorders in the elderly are ignored because their onset is so slow as to go unnoticed: Parkinsonism, dementia and cancer to mention but a few. The presenting symptoms of many disorders are different in the elderly to those in other age groups, becoming much vaguer with age. The elderly often tell their doctor they just feel unwell — and can only offer symptoms such as tiredness or weakness — making it extremely difficult, and time-consuming to establish the cause of the illness. Faced with this situation, the doctor may be tempted to ascribe the symptoms to old age rather than to disease, and perhaps give the patient a tablet (iron, vitamins and tranquillisers being popular choices) in the hope that the symptoms will go away.

Clearly the elderly present enormous difficulties to the medical profession when deciding the appropriate course of action.

STRATEGIES FOR INVESTIGATION

Geriatric medicine is probably the most general form of internal medicine. It is also a specialization. It requires both a knowledge of all tests and treatments used in general medicine, and an understanding of how they must be adapted and interpreted when administered to the elderly.

As far as medical testing goes, a doctor must bear the following in mind when presented with an elderly patient:

1.   Many old people will find it difficult or impossible to submit to certain tests, so a doctor must be aware of more appropriate alternatives. They may also refuse, from understandable embarrassment, to provide specimens of urine or faeces.

2.   Since the symptoms may well be very general, a doctor must know which tests are most likely to provide clues to diagnosis, in order to avoid an unnecessary battery of tests.

3.   Test results can be affected by:

●   **changes in physiology due to age: a normal result for a 65 year old may be different from that for a 25 year old.**

●   **the presence of more than one pathology**

For the purpose of medical testing, the elderly can be grouped into three categories:

●   **those without symptoms for whom health screening may be appropriate;**

●   **those arriving at their doctor's surgery or at hospital with vague symptoms that do not suggest an obvious diagnosis;**

●   **those with suspected disorders that need to be confirmed.**

HEALTH SCREENING FOR THE ELDERLY

If elderly people do not come to a doctor for help, should a doctor assume they are healthy and in no need of medical assistance? Doctors are divided about the appropriateness of preventative medicine — *screening* (the search for asymptomatic disease) and *case-finding* (identifying and managing previously unreported problems) — in geriatrics.

SCREENING

In the past 20 years the following have been proposed as screening tests for use in elderly populations:

- chest X-ray

- urea and electrolytes

- haemoglobin levels

- erythrocyte sedimentation rate

- whole blood count

- culture of mid-stream urine specimen

- urinalysis

- thyroid status

- faecal occult blood

- tonometry (measuring pressure in different parts of the body)

- cervical cancer screening for women over 65

However, there is no evidence that if routinely applied to a whole population of healthy elderly people, any of these tests shorten the duration of any disease, or prevent loss of functional ability or the need for long-stay care.

It has also been impossible to identify 'at risk' groups who might benefit from screening. When the Medical Research Council Sociology Unit in Aberdeen ran a study of risk profiles in the elderly nothing conclusive was achieved. Their groupings: over 80 years, recently widowed, never married, living alone, socially isolated, without children, in poor economic circumstances, recently discharged from hospital, having recent change of dwelling and divorced/separated, were not sensitive enough for routine use in primary care.

One group for whom screening has been shown to be effective is those old people thought to require residential care. One screening study of a 100 such people resulted in 32 being placed more appropriately than in the old people's home they had been thought to need.

CASE-FINDING

Various studies looking at case-finding have demonstrated that elderly people do have many unreported problems. But what constitutes a problem depends on your point of view. To the doctor a problem is a situation or condition that poses an appropriate challenge to his or her skills; to an old person a problem is a difficulty, but not necessarily one for which medical help should be sought.

An old person may not seek help for a variety of reasons:

- because s/he cannot — through immobility or inability to communicate;

- because s/he does not realize medical intervention is necessary.

In these situations, case-finding is appropriate, although may be disappointing to the old person if the problem then turns out to be insoluble.

Some old people prefer not to go to their doctor, perhaps through fear of institutionalization, dashed hopes or invasion of privacy. These fears may not always be conscious and there is therefore an ethical problem for the case finders — should they challenge the old person's statement and attempt to change their decision or accept it and leave them alone? This problem is most easily avoided if the case finder is a GP, well known to the old person, particularly is that GP is prepared to

- visit the person more than once — as the admission of a problem may only be made on the second or third visit, and

- assure the person that the objective of the exercise is to keep the old person in their own home if that is what (s)he wants.

Challenging an old person's view that they are 'all right' is not a sign of disrespect, but if after such a challenge they still refuse help, their wishes should be respected.

A health centre in East Oxford have actually introduced a simple, inexpensive case-finding system to monitor the elderly patients in their practice. They decided to follow up those people aged over 75 who had had no contact with the primary care team during one year. The doctors participating felt that the programme did strengthen the relationship between the primary care team and the patient — a relationship that is extremely important in encouraging early referral, compliance and appropriate use of the health services. They therefore concluded that the project was worth while and should be explored by other health centres.

DIAGNOSING AN OLD PERSON WITH VAGUE SYMPTOMS OF ILL HEALTH

INTERVIEW

As with any diagnosis, the first step will be an interview at which a medical history will be taken, followed by a physical examination. While elderly patients are just as capable of giving an account of their problems as other age groups, the following problems can limit and disrupt communication between the doctor and patients:

- dementia (in 10% of the elderly),

- impaired hearing (in 22% of the elderly),

- visual handicap (in 15% of the elderly).

If any of the above apply, the interview will take much longer. There is really no excuse if the doctor is impatient, and (s)he should always speak clearly facing the patient, if necessary, writing down the questions. Doctors sometimes ask for someone who knows the elderly person to be present at the interview. This can help the doctor establish information about capacity before the onset of present illness. Past medical records also provide extremely valuable information and in many cases investigations previously carried out need not be repeated, saving time and money. It is certainly worth mentioning any recent investigations in case the doctor does not have access to all the records.

Health care of the elderly, perhaps more than any other age group, is influenced by the social support system available to them. So a doctor will try and find out information about the following:

- standards of care and help available at home

- factors contributing to illness: malnutrition (alcohol), dehydration, neglect and poor habits, adverse drug reactions

- domestic impediments to resettlement e.g. stairs after strokes

- relationships with friends and relatives

- supporting services — the need; those already in use; availability of others

It is important for the doctor to be given as much information as possible on medication history and to insist (s)he checks it as elderly people are specifically vulnerable to the adverse effects of medication and, therefore, iatrogenic (doctor induced) diseases.

PHYSICAL EXAMINATION

Before performing a physical examination the doctor should seek permission. If necessary a doctor can make a decision and recommend treatment from a provisional diagnosis without a physical examination, so no-one should feel pressurized to agree to one.

During the examination the doctor will first try to get an impression of general health — skin, hair, temperature and so on. Special consideration will be given to the detection of

- thyroid, breast and cervical cancer

- occult bleeding

- hypertension

- postural hypotension

- disease in the oral cavity that may impair nutritional status

- wax impaction in the ears that may limit hearing

- serious auditory or opthalmic disorders

- bowel function and the possible presence of varying degrees of urinary incontinence and sleep disturbance

- postural stability — in view of the high prevalence and serious consequences of falls in the elderly

- hypothermia

The elderly person may then be asked some questions to assess mental state. This is because dementia, the chronic, often progressive loss of intellectual function, is a major cause of disability in the elderly. Certain forms are treatable, so the test can be of great help. Treatable forms of dementia include

- acute confusion due to toxic, infective, metabolic and deficiency states, and

- certain depression or persecutory states.

Primary dementias such as Alzheimer's disease are not treatable, but the knowledge that the condition exists will help everyone concerned, relatives and doctor make plans for the future.

The sorts of questions that are asked of the patient include:

1. How old are you?

2. When is your birthday (month and date)?

3. Address to remember (to be repeated by patient at end of test)

4. What place are we in?

5. What is the year now?

6. Recognition of two people either by name (e.g. relative) or by appearance (e.g. nurse)

7. What is the time now (to the nearest hour)?

8. Have we a Queen or King? What is his/her name?

9. In what year did the Second World War start?

10. Count backwards from 20 to one.

These questions can be varied according to ethnic origins. Anything less than 10 out of 10 is considered to be abnormal. The test is for the presence of confusion, not its cause.

Such questions can be considered offensive by some patients, who may nevertheless be quite confused. An alternative, although not validated, is the 'four sets'. The patient is asked to name as many animals, flowers, colours, and vegetables as possible, and is stopped after 10 names in each set. If the subject 'dries up', encouraging remarks can be made by the doctor. A total score of less than 30 suggests significant mental impairment.

If there is mental impairment it is then necessary to establish the cause. At least half and perhaps as many as 70% of patients suffering from dementia have Alzheimer's disease.

Efforts are under way to improve the sensitivity and specificity of CT scans and EEG evaluations of patients with Alzheimer's disease. Until now CT scans have been unable to provide definitive diagnostic information, often not distinguishing patients with the disease from unaffected individuals. Their use has been limited to the exclusion of potentially treatable conditions. EEG can show clear difference between those patients with, and those without Alzheimer's disease.

The range of other diagnostic tests a doctor may employ in diagnosis is similar to other age groups; some were listed under the screening section, other commonly used diagnostic procedures include:

- blood sample(s) to measure
  - haemoglobin, white blood count and mean corpuscular volume
  - plasma sodium, potassium, urea and glucose
  - serum C-reactive protein levels
  - serum albumin levels

- blood culture (where there is any suspicion of bacterial infection)

- X-ray of abdomen (taken to include both hip joints)

- test of mental function

- core temperature — particularly where hypothermia is suspected

- aspiration or collections of fluid (especially pleural or joint effusions) to look for evidence of infection, including tuberculosis

- ECG

CONFIRMATION OF SUSPECTED COMMON DISORDERS OF THE ELDERLY

Degenerative and locomotor disorders are pre-eminent in the elderly, and the outstanding physical limitations in old age are imposed by:

- cardiovascular disease

- arthritis (osteoarthrosis, rheumatoid disease)

- neuro-muscular disorders (Parkinsonism, motor neurone disease)

- cancer

- pulmonary infections

- thrombo-embolism

- mental disorders

RESPIRATORY DISORDERS

These are very common and important in the elderly, causing both acute illness and chronic disability. Diagnosis depends on very accurate clinical observation of the limitations of radiology in the elderly and the impracticability and difficulty of interpretation of many tests of respiratory function. Five important factors are

- smoking history

- cough (+analysis of sputum)

- breathlessness

- chest pain

- wheezing/effect of weather on chest.

Age changes in the lungs themselves as well as weakness of the accessory muscles of respiration mean that physical signs may be less evident in the elderly.

CARDIOVASCULAR DISORDERS

These are also very common in old age. Proper interpretation of the major symptoms of cardiac disease is particularly difficult in the elderly because two important symptoms, cardiac pain and dypsnoea, are frequently modified, and a third — oedema — is only relatively infrequently due to cardiac disease. Clinical examination is much more likely to provide answers than radiology or electrocardiography. These investigations often either confirm what is already known from the clinical examination, or tend to confuse the issue by introducing irrelevancies.

Similar tests are carried out on the elderly as for younger cardiovascular patients. However, the results must be interpreted by a geriatrics specialist because of the variation in normal values.

GASTROINTESTINAL SYSTEM

Symptoms and signs of gastrointestinal disease are similar in all age groups, but sometimes such symptoms are due to disturbances outside of the gastrointestinal system in the aged. This can cause problems with diagnosis. Diagnosis in the elderly relies heavily on interview and clinical examination.

The dental state and whether or not false teeth are used should be recorded. Physical signs in the acute abdomen in the elderly patient are often hard to elicit. The absence of bowel sound may be the only indication that something is amiss. Constipation is common; and diarrhoea and vomiting are always sinister in old age.

Elderly patients will undergo the same battery of tests as any other group, with whatever modifications are necessary to accommodate the changes and disabilities associated with age. Special care will be taken with the interpretation of the results.

ENDOCRINE/METABOLIC DISORDERS

Diabetes and disorders of the thyroid gland are common in old age. Standard tests are used, but with different 'normal' ranges.

GENITO-URINARY DISORDERS

Urinary symptoms are very common, especially nocturnal frequency and incontinence of urine. The most important examination is palpation of bladder. In old men the doctor should examine the external genitalia. In old women a vaginal examination may be attempted if possible. A cervical smear for women over 65 may be recommended, to test for cancer.

There are considerable limitations when testing the elderly for genito-urinary disorders. These are largely imposed by the sensitivity of the patient, but also the physiological changes that have inevitably taken place.

NERVOUS DISORDERS

Many changes take place in the nervous system as a result of age-ing, and these need to be taken into account in evaluating neu-rological disorders. A simple example is the reduction of knee jerk response with age.

At the initial interview, the doctor will ask a lot of questions. It is often impossible to discover from the history what in fact is the precise nature of the turns, blackouts or falls. Under these circumstances the doctor will attempt to demonstrate possible mechanisms, such as postural drop in blood pressure, by observing the patient while walking; and if necessary a period of hospital observation in an attempt to provide witnesses for the symptoms.

Where possible, the patient should be asked to stand so that balance and gait can be assessed. Minor motor, co-ordination and sensory disturbances often only become apparent when this is done. Some perceptual disorders as a result of a stroke are often not noticed even though they cause considerable disability. So the old person may be asked to try and copy something drawn by the doctor. Other similar tests will be performed to help predict functional independence and survival after a stroke.

The full battery of other diagnostic techniques for nervous dis-orders will also be employed.

MENTAL FUNCTION

See under Physical examination, above.

BONE DISEASE

The same battery of diagnostic tests as for other age groups is employed. Special attention is given to the diagnosis of osteopo-rosis in elderly women. There are several different tests that meas-ure the density of bone, although there is no one absolutely accurate test. They include

- CT scans

- nuclear scanning

- measuring calcium in the blood and urine

- phosphorus and alkaline phosphatase tests

- measurement of pharthyroid hormone levels and oestrogen testing

- bone biopsy

SKIN DISEASES

The state of the skin should be noted in any physical examination.

HAEMATOLOGICAL DISORDERS

In order to test accurately for iron deficiency a doctor has to be aware that levels vary in old people depending on their health.

DRUG INDUCED PROBLEMS

Measurement of the plasma concentrations of certain drugs of clinical importance in the elderly can help diagnose both toxicity and also whether recommended drug therapy has been followed by the patient.

LOCOMOTOR SYSTEM

Abnormalities are common and often very important since they limit mobility. The state of the toe nails should always be recorded. Opportunities should be taken to observe the patient getting out of a chair or bed and during walking — often this reveals that the locomotor problem is due to pain, weakness, stiffness or instability.

IMMUNE SYSTEM

Ageing is associated with a deterioration in the immediate and delayed response of the immune system to injury or infection. Practical implications of this are that the signs and symptoms of acute illness are often masked.

CONCLUSION

Old age brings with it many medical problems — some of which can be relieved, others that cannot. Before agreeing to any examinations or investigations, an elderly patient should discuss with their doctor what can be done for the condition under investigation, should the test results prove positive. If the answer is very little, the patient, or their relatives, should question the value of undergoing the proposed test(s).

Chapter 6

WOMEN

More and more tests are now available to women making it difficult to know which is the safest and most effective. Regional variations in resources mean that the most appropriate test may not be readily available in your local hospital or clinic. This chapter tries to set the record straight!

DISORDERS OF THE BREAST

Breast cancer, both benign (ie non-cancerous) and malignant (cancerous), is extremely common in women and breast cancer is the leading cause of death for women between 35 and 44.

The causes of breast disease are unclear, so prevention is problematic, but it has been shown that earlier treatment of breast cancer does increase survival and improve the woman's quality of life, as compared to late treatment. There is therefore a need for effective screening and diagnosis.

The experts have found it difficult to identify 'at risk groups' and it has been suggested by some that all women should be treated as at appreciable risk from breast cancer. Likely risk factors include:

- cancer in one breast

- no children or late first child

- age

- incidence of benign breast disease

- incidence of breast cancer in mother's family

- early first period

- late onset of menopause

- having had DES (diethylstilboestrol)

- obesity (particularly if also diabetic)

The Government, in announcing a National Breast Screening Programme in 1987, took up the recommendation of the Forrest Report of screening women over 50 and under 64.

SCREENING FOR BREAST DISEASE: BREAST SELF-EXAMINATION (BSE)

90% of all breast lumps (benign or malignant) are discovered by women themselves. BSE is therefore encouraged.

Most lumps are not malignant and all breasts become naturally lumpy in the week before a period. Regular BSE should detect any abnormal changes of the breast.

What you are looking for:

- unusual lump(s)

- unusual pain or discomfort

- changes in the skin of the breast, e.g. puckering or dimpling

- unusual drawing back or turning in of the nipple

- persistent puslike or foul-smelling discharge from either nipple

- skin trouble on or around the nipple

- swelling of the upper arm

- unusual changes in the size or shape of the breast or one breast being unusually higher or lower than the other

- enlarges lymphatic nodes under the armpit

HOW TO DO A BREAST EXAMINATION

Ideally a BSE should be attempted regularly once a month — just after a period if you are menstruating, or on the same day each month if you are not. There are several techniques for BSE, so find one you are happy with and stick with it. Some women find BSE easier in the bath or shower; others prefer lying in bed. However, the basic steps include:

Observation: stand in front of a mirror with your arms by your side, then with your hands on your hips and your elbows as far back as possible, and then with your arms straight up over your head.

Palpation: first while you are standing in front of the mirror and then while lying on your back with one arm (the arm on the same side as the breast being examined) behind your head and using the rib cage for resistance, press the fingertips gently but firmly into the breast tissue, using a circular motion from the outside in towards the nipple, until the entire breast has been palpated. Pay special attention to the area between the nipple and the armpit, which is the most common location of tumours. Squeeze the nipple to observe whether there is any discharge.

THE VALUE OF BSE

Retrospective studies of BSE have produced mixed results, with some studies showing an association of BSE with earlier detection and others not. No prospective study has been done with mortality as an outcome. A trial is underway in the UK comparing BSE both with a screening programme of clinical breast examination (CBE) and mammography and with no screening programme at all; but the results will not be available for many years.

As currently practised BSE accuracy (sensitivity and specificity) is not as good as the combination of clinical breast examination and mammography. And little is known about the effects of BSE on the anxiety levels among the women — for example, why do 90 to 99% of US women know of BSE but only 14 to 40% actually practise it? The Forrest Report recommended that teaching BSE should not be included in the screening programme in this country.

To give the World Health Organisation the last word "there is insufficient evidence that BSE as applied to date is effective in reducing mortality from breast cancer; therefore BSE screening programmes are not at present recommended as public health policy, although there is equally insufficient evidence to change them where they already exist".

SCREENING FOR BREAST DISEASE: MASS SCREENING

In mass screening for breast cancer, large numbers of women are involved who have no disease and would not be having the examination were it not for the availability of the screening service. The detection process should therefore be quick, safe, readily available, economical and acceptable to the women being screened. It should also be able to detect cancer at a stage when it can be treated.

In the past breast screening took the following form:

Interview   to establish ethnic background, parity, menstrual and breast history with the aim of getting clues as to increased risk.

Clinical breast examination (CBE)   by physician or trained paramedic. The doctor will examine you much in the same way as you examine yourself and should be as gentle. Your doctor may include examinations of your abdomen to feel whether or not the liver is enlarged. Both breasts should always be examined.

Teaching BSE (see above)

Mammography. This is a standard X-ray of the breast. The aim of mammography is to discover cancer in its earliest stages or to confirm the surgeon's view that no carcinoma (tumour) is present. (See Chapter 2 for details). The radiologist will ask you

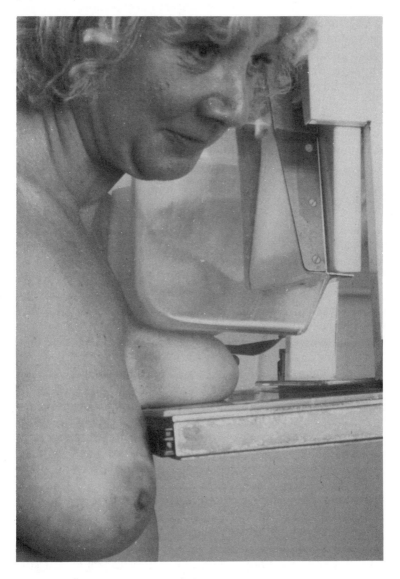

Figure 21. A woman undergoing X-ray mammography.

to pose in a variety of positions so that your breasts can be photographed from different angles.

Do not use any perfumes or deodorants on the day of the mammogram as these can obscure the mammograms. You should also tell the doctor if you are pregnant or breast-feeding.

The radiation dose is now less than 0.1 rad to the mid breast per complete examination. A recent study estimates that less than 1% of all cases of breast cancer result from diagnostic radiography such as mammograms. Some doctors still use xeromammography which uses the usual X-ray equipment with xerox process. The radiation dose is six times that of modern film screen combinations.

However, the new screening service will now only provide a mammography with no clinical examination.

THE VALUE OF MAMMOGRAPHY

Early detection of breast cancer leads to an increased chance of survival particularly of women over 50. The NHS is to make available screening for women aged between 50 and 64 every three years. It is hoped to save one third of the current 15,000 deaths a year.

However, there is still, at best, a false negative rate of 10%. Errors are numerous, but not so great as to diminish the value of the examination. Many benign tumours are removed because they appear 'suspicious' on mammograms, but few cancers are missed.

In Britain there is nothing to prevent anyone setting up a mobile breast screening clinic as long as they employ a qualified radiologist. Many women are taking advantage of the service. Unfortunately the standard of diagnosis is often extremely inaccurate due to substandard equipment or sub-standard technicians. Most important — don't go to any unit or answer a private advertisement, without checking it out. The private sector may provide screening, but the best person to recommend the clinic is your doctor.

It is not only the private sector that is providing a poor service; many NHS units also practise with a similar lack of expertise. Hospital machines in some areas are so obsolete that they produce the same poor quality film.

Quality control is urgently needed and it seems that the Government will license out-patient units in the private sector so checks can be made on their activities.

DIAGNOSIS OF BREAST DISEASE

If you find a lump in the course of a self examination it is not necessarily cancer. It is most likely to be a fluid filled cyst or a fibroidenoma (benign tumour). If after one menstrual cycle the lump is still there, consult your doctor. His/her approach will depend on your age and the type of lump found. Lumps in the breasts of older women are treated as being malignant until proved otherwise. This can be unnecessarily worrying but it does at least ensure that you will usually see a specialist (usually a surgeon) very quickly — sometimes within 36 to 48 hours. You will almost certainly have a mammography if you have not already had one. Other imaging techniques include the following (see Chapter 2 for details):

Ultrasound: this technique is being used more and more. For example, in Australia it is routinely used with symptomatic women under 30 to reduce the frequency of X-ray mammography.

Currently its accuracy does not compare with X-ray mammography, particularly for minimal lesions. It is expected that there will come a time when ultrasound's accuracy will be equal to or greater than X-ray.

Thermography: this is certainly a non-evasive technique for detecting cancer, but its accuracy is not yet as good as X-ray.

Transillumination: another non-invasive test. Transillumination can differentiate between a cyst and a solid mass. It is approaching the diagnostic accuracy of mammography.

Nuclear magnetic resonance/imaging: this is proving to be an effective way to distinguish harmless lumps from those that must be removed. At present it is an extremely expensive technique, but in the future will become less expensive simpler and more available and promises to be an extremely sensitive method for early detection of cancer. It is non-invasive and non-hazardous.

Digital radiography: this utilizes high-efficiency X-ray detectors which can reduce X-ray doses well below that of film/screen and xeromammography units, probably to the level of yearly background radiation.

Radionuclide studies: these techniques are useful for highlighting tumours and increasingly being used.

DIAGNOSTIC TECHNIQUES IN BREAST DISORDERS

Needle aspiration: if the mass disappears after withdrawal of the fluid, it was a cyst and the problem is now solved. If the mass is still present, it may have to be biopsied if no other cyst is found elsewhere in the breast. If the fluid is blood-tinged, a biopsy will probably be recommended as it may contain cancer cells from a cancer in the cyst.

Biopsy:

● needle biopsy

● open biopsy of either all or some of the lump

Both types of biopsy take about 30 to 40 minutes. After the operation your breast will feel tender and achy for about a week. If the pain does not subside and is accompanied by fever, redness or discharge, see your doctor. Because there are now techniques available to analyse the biopsy sample while you are still under anaesthetic (see Chapter 2) the surgeon has the option of performing further surgery, such as a mastectomy before you come round. You should therefore discuss with your surgeon the options **before** the operation and read any forms you are given to sign very carefully. It is inexcusable for a woman to wake up from what she thought was a biopsy and find she has also undergone a mastectomy.

DISORDERS OF THE URINOGENITAL SYSTEM

This includes all conditions related to organs and tissues concerned with excretion and reproduction. These are anatomically closely associated — particularly so in women.

PHYSICAL EXAMINATION

Self-examination: this can be done with a hand held mirror, a torch, KY jelly and a speculum (available from most chemists). As with breast examination the object is to build up a picture of what is normal for you through regular examination and therefore to detect any abnormalities. Do not attempt a self examination if you are pregnant, have just given birth, or after gynaecological surgery. This is because there is an increased risk of infection. Before examining yourself, empty your bladder, then find a comfortable bed or couch and sit or lie down with your knees bent and feet well apart. Prop yourself up comfortably with cushions. Practise using the speculum before insertion, then lubricate it and gently insert — much as you would a tampon. Once the speculum is in place move the light and mirror until you can see into the vagina and possibly the cervix. The cervix can be difficult to locate because it is often off to one side. To remove the speculum, keep it open and slowly pull it straight out. Always wash and dry the speculum well after use.

Clinical examination: the following internal (pelvic) examination should be carried out at a family planning, VD or antenatal clinic in addition to your local surgery, and should not take more than 5 to 10 minutes including a cervical smear (see on). All women should have a regular check up, but if you have any condition that might put you at risk, it is even more important. An internal pelvic examination is the only way doctors can discover an ovarian tumour which is another forceful argument for regular check ups. A team at King's College Hospital in London are working on an ultrasound scanning technique for screening women for ovarian cancer which they hope will one day become a standard screening technique in the same way as cervical smears.

The clinical examination should include:

Inspection of the external genitals (vulva): to check for

- abnormalities,

- irritations,

- discoloration,

- unusual vaginal discharge.

The doctor may also examine the anterior wall of the vagina for loss of bladder wall support (cystoceles), and rectocele (a bulge of the rectum into the vagina), by pressing on the back wall of the vagina (towards the rectum) and ask you to bear down. (S)he will also look for

- a loss of urine when you cough (stress incontinence)

- pus in the Skene's glands (which are at the entrance of the urinary opening)

- presence of Bartholin's cysts, and

- the strength of pelvic-floor and abdominal muscles.

Speculum examination: A speculum is a hinged, bivalved instrument that spreads the walls of the vagina exposing the cervix. It should be gently inserted into the vagina — and warmed beforehand if metal! A cervical smear will be taken at this point (see on).

Bimanual vaginal examination: The doctor inserts two gloved fingers into the vagina where (s)he can feel the tip of the cervix. The cervix has an opening at the centre of it. With his/her hand pressing on your abdomen, (s)he can outline the contours of the cervix, uterus, tubes and ovaries — feeling for any enlargement, irregular shape or tenderness. This is a rather uncomfortable examination which is unfortunately only made easier by relaxing, something that does not come easily under such circumstances!

Recto-vaginal examination: Finally the doctor will insert one finger into the vagina and one into the rectum in order to feel for certain abnormalities of the rectum as polyps and get information about the tome and alignment of the pelvic organs. You may feel as though you are having a bowel movement as the doctor withdraws his/her finger, but in fact this will not happen.

CERVICAL (PAP) SMEARS

A cervical smear is a screening technique that shows if there is any disease at the neck of the womb (cervix) which might develop into cancer.

Regular cervical smears do lead to the discovery and early treatment of invasive cancer of the cervix — often, but not always resulting in a cure, but only if the screening programme is properly organized and screens those most at risk — as in Sweden, Finland and Iceland where there has been a significant fall in mortality from cervical carcinoma. In the UK there has only been a small decrease in mortality, and in younger age groups there has been a worrying increase in the number of deaths. The problems with cervical screening in the UK are in large measure due to an expensive medical technique being introduced without prior evaluation, and before suitable arrangements for the administration of the service had been agreed. A new lobby group 'Women Against Cervical Cancer' has recently been set up to help improve the service in this country — this is certainly a welcome development.

The Department of Health recommends that screening should start two years after becoming sexually active and should be repeated every five years. Other countries recommend a three year recall and the American College of Obstetrics and Gynaecology, a yearly recall. Certain groups are screened more frequently — on a yearly or even six months basis; they include those who have:

- had a previous abnormal smear

- been on the pill for more than five years

- a history or presence of vaginal and/or vulval warts

- partners who have or have had a history of penile or anal warts

- partners who have or have had many sexual partners

- or have had many sexual partners themselves

- a history of heavy smoking

HAVING A CERVICAL SMEAR

You can get a cervical smear at a family planning clinic, or local health centre. Some GPs also offer a screening service. The test is free. It can be carried out by a doctor or a trained paramedic.

If you are menstruating, the best time to have a smear is mid cycle, because the presence of blood can interfere with the test results. You should tell the person doing the test if you

- are on any medication — as some do affect the test results

- might be pregnant

- are taking any contraceptive pill.

In the US, doctors suggest that you should avoid douching, having a bath and even sexual intercourse 24 hours before the test as all can affect the outcome. You will feel more comfortable during the test if you empty your bladder beforehand.

You will be asked to remove all your clothing below the waist and to lie on an examining table. You will either have your feet raised and supported by stirrups or will be asked to bend your knees and open your legs. A vaginal speculum is inserted and the examiner then reaches into the vagina with a swab and/or spatula and takes at least three specimens which are treated, and then sent to the laboratory for analysis by a trained technician.

The accuracy of cytodiagnosis depends on the quality of the smear and the way in which it was obtained as well as on the skill and experience of the cytologist. Up to 10% of all smears have to be discarded because they were made by untrained doctors or nurses. One of the problems has been the standardization of the terminology used to describe the smear results. The British Society for Clinical Cytology have now recommended a standard terminology and it is hoped that this will be implemented.

As with breast screening, there are private laboratories offering a cervical screening service. The London Programme early in 1987 put one to the test. They added 22 clearly visible cancerous smears to the normal delivery of 800 smears to the laboratory. Five were missed, three of which were of serious disease. Five cases of serious disease were passed off as mild abnormality. Therefore 10 out of 22 positive smears were misdiagnosed.

Profit, not the patient motivates these laboratories. Technicians work longer hours to complete quotas, often with no pathologist in residence and little information on the patients whose smears they are sorting. There are already 40 such clinics in the UK and Government is considering farming out NHS smears to private laboratories for analysis. In principle there is nothing wrong with this — but only if there is legislation to safeguard standards of practice.

NHS doctors are also guilty of misdiagnosis on a grand scale as was recently evidenced in Liverpool, where 911 women were wrongly diagnosed. There is therefore a real need for an over-haul of the system if women are to be persuaded that having a cervical smear is good for their physical, or indeed emotional wellbeing.

GETTING THE RESULTS

The time interval before the results are available varies enormously from region to region. In the US results are usually ready after 1 to 2 weeks. In this country you can sometimes expect to wait months, even if your last test was positive. Some clinics notify all women screened of their results, usually by post. Others only notify those whose smears were positive — leaving it open to ques-tion whether not receiving a letter means your test was negative or just lost! Even if you do receive a letter it may not be forth-coming with your result. It may simply ask you to come for a repeat smear, without telling you why, leaving you wondering "have I got cancer?" The only advice the authors can give is that you check with the person who did the smear when the results will be ready, and how you can obtain them.

WHAT HAPPENS IF YOUR CERVICAL SMEAR IS POSITIVE?

The action taken will depend on whether the smear showed signs of cancer or not. Generally, if the abnormality was due to infec-tion, the infection will be treated and a repeat smear taken after two to six months. A repeat smear will also be taken, if any other non-cancerous abnormality were found. Further action will be taken if the second smear is positive. The table below shows the pattern of investigation following a positive smear.

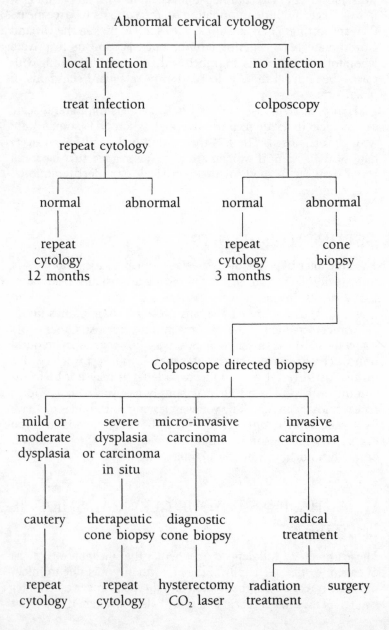

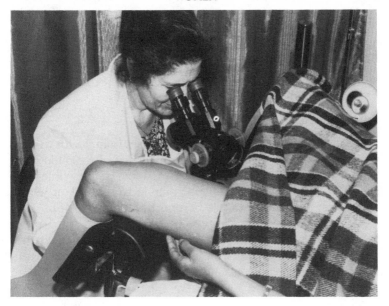

Figure 22. A doctor examining a woman's cervix using a colposcope.

COLPOSCOPY

Colposcopy is used for the further study of women whose cervical smear is reported as positive (see Chapter 2 for details of scoping techniques). Most clinics will refer you for one after a second positive smear. Women who have taken, or whose mothers have taken, DES (diethylstilboestrol) may also be referred for a colposcopy to monitor the health of their vagina, because of the increased risk of vaginal cancer. Examination using a colposcope may be enough to diagnose early invasive cervical carcinoma, although usually a biopsy is taken from the worst areas to confirm the diagnosis before undertaking local destructive therapy of a pre-invasive lesion.

Colposcopies are usually done on an out-patient basis in a hospital by specially trained clinicians. The test should not be painful although women do report mild cramping. It is certainly uncomfortable. It usually takes about 15 minutes to carry out. There will probably be some bleeding and/or discharge for about a week afterwards, but there should be no heavy bleeding, fever or pain. If there is, notify your doctor. If a biopsy was performed the cervix will need time to heal so it is better to avoid sexual intercourse and douching for a week.

Discuss the results of the colposcopy with the clinician and if a biopsy was taken, ask when the results will be available and how you should go about getting them.

CERVICAL BIOPSY

The decision to recommend a biopsy varies from doctor to doctor, but in general should only be recommended where colposcopy cannot give a sufficiently accurate assessment of the whole field at risk to enable a safe therapeutic plan to be evolved, or where abnormal epithelium extends beyond the limit of vision.

Multiple punch biopsy: This a fairly simple operation carried out on an out-patient basis without any anaesthetic. Small pieces of tissue are removed for examination. There may be some bleeding and/or discharge for a week or two after the operation.

Cone biopsy: This is done under anaesthetic in a hospital. A small cone of tissue is removed from the cervix. In some cases cone biopsy serves as treatment too as all the diseased tissue may be removed during the biopsy. There are considerable dangers involved in having a cone biopsy: extensive bleeding, infection and problems with later pregnancies — due to the fact that the cervix is no longer able to dilate naturally. For this reason it is not usually carried out on a pregnant woman until after delivery. It may also interfere with fertility.

OTHER TECHNIQUES USED IN THE INVESTIGATION OF UROGENITAL DISORDERS IN WOMEN

Endometrial biopsy: If your doctor suspects there is something wrong with your endometrium he will recommend an endometrial biopsy. A biopsy can establish why

● there has been a change in menstrual bleeding pattern.

● there is bleeding in women who have already gone through menopause.

● a woman has not been able to conceive.

Endometrial biopsies can be carried out without anaesthetic, in which case you may experience some cramping during the biopsy. Alternatively you may undergo *Dilation and Curettage* (D & C) which is performed in hospital under general anaesthetic. Prior to a D & C tell the doctor if you are pregnant or are rhesus negative, and your doctor should check that the operation will be performed in the correct phase of your cycle (if infertility is being investigated).

The operation involves one day in hospital followed by a check up by the GP six weeks later. There may be some bleeding and it will take a few days to get over the after effects of the anaesthetic.

Laparoscopy: This is a minor operation in which your doctor inserts a slender light containing a telescope into your abdomen to look at your pelvic organs and abdominal organs (see Chapter 2 for details of scoping techniques). Common diagnostic reasons for laparoscopy include:

- infertility

- primary or secondary amenorrhea

- ectopic pregnancy

- undiagnosed pelvic pain

- pelvic adhesions

- endometriosis

- twisting of an ovary

- ruptured ovarian cyst

- undiagnosed masses

- uterine perforation

- internal haemorrhage

- perforation by IUD (or coil)

Laparoscopy is usually performed under general anaesthetic, although surgery can be done under spinal or epidural anaesthetic. Preparation, surgery and recovery take an average of four to five hours. It is usually an out-patient operation and is generally only an in-patient operation if you have medical problems or complications. Recovery is quick — usually less than one to two days.

Culdocentesis: This test is usually done to diagnose ectopic pregnancy or tubal infections. It is performed in hospital by a physician and an assistant without anaesthetic. You will be asked to walk or sit up for a short time before the test begins to encourage the drainage of fluids into the lower abdomen. You will then be asked to strip from the waist down, and lie with your knees or heels resting in stirrups. First a pelvic examination will be performed then the physician will grasp the cervix with a tenaculum, lift it slightly and insert a long thin needle through the vaginal wall below the uterus, withdrawing a sample up into the syringe. If no fluid is found, a second or third attempt may be made at a slightly different angle. You may have an uncomfortable pulling sensation as the cervix is grasped and there is a brief sharp pain when the needle is inserted. If fresh blood is found, emergency surgery may be needed. If an infection is present, a culture of the fluid can suggest the appropriate treatment.

COMMON VAGINAL AND URINARY TRACT INFECTIONS IN WOMEN

Vaginitis: This is an inflammation of the vagina and vulva. In order to make a diagnosis your doctor will perform a pelvic examination, and take a sample of vaginal discharge. This is then examined for fungus (yeast), parasites (trichomonas) and bacterial (hemophilus or gardnerella) infections. You should ask your doctor when the results of these analyses will be ready.

Pelvic inflammatory disease (PID):   This refers to a group of pelvic infections. A sample of cervical discharge will be taken and then cultured to establish which organism is present. PID has the same symptoms as ectopic pregnancy and endometriosis; a pregnancy test is also usually performed. Again, you should ask your doctor when the results will be available.

Cystitis: This is an inflammation and/or infection of the bladder. To diagnose it, a urine sample will be taken for analysis in order to find out which bacteria is involved. This is important as treatments vary according to the type of bacteria present. You should ask when the results will be ready.

Endometritis: This is an inflammation of the uterine lining. Diagnosis is made by a bi-manual pelvic examination, and then a sample of cervical discharge is taken for analysis. Do check when the results will be ready.

Yeast infections (thrush): These infections occur in the vagina, so to make a diagnosis a sample of vaginal discharge will be taken. This is mainly to ensure that the infection is thrush and not any other type of infection.

CONTRACEPTION

Whether you go to a family planning clinic, well woman clinic or your own GP, you should receive the following check up before being prescribed your choice of contraception:

- Interview: name, address, age, marital status (not always), medical history,

- Weight

- Blood pressure

- Internal examination by doctor

- Discussion with doctor of possible methods.

If you chose an IUD or coil, a cervical smear, and VD tests should be done as well. If insertion is not carried out during a period, a pregnancy test should also be done. In many clinics these precautions are not taken in advance and evidence of infection may only come to light at your next examination. If you choose a diaphragm a nurse will need to measure your upper vagina to get the right size of diaphragm for you.

INFERTILITY

One in eight couples have difficulty conceiving. However, most infertility problems are minor and need only fairly straightforward treatment for conception to occur. Women are marginally more likely to have a fertility problem than men, although 30% of infertility is caused by men alone. In 20% of cases it is both partners that are contributing to the problem.

The first step is to go with your partner to your GP. (S)he may do some simple tests, and then decide if you should be referred preferably to a fertility clinic where specialized facilities are available. At the clinic you and your partner will undergo a series of tests usually over a period of three to five months. The following tests may be carried out, the order varying according to your particular problems and the policy of the clinic.

INFERTILITY TESTS FOR WOMEN

Test	Cycle day	Performed by	What test is looking for
1. Tests of ovulation			
basal body temp	throughout	yourself	ovulation (temperature rises before) right time to have intercourse
blood tests	24	laboratory	progesterone level rises before ovulation high prolactin level can stop ovulation antibodies

Test	Cycle day	Performer by	What test is looking for
endometrium biopsy	19	doctor (general anaesthetic)	ovulation state of uterus
observation of ovaries via laparoscopy	second half of cycle	doctor (general anaesthetic)	condition of ovaries
mucus quality: using post-coital	at ovulation	doctor	live vigorous sperm in mucus incompatibility with partner amount/thick-ness
observation	throughout	you or doctor	
2. *Test of reproductive system*			
blowing tubes (insufflation)	any time	doctor	any blockages
HSG* (Hystero-salpingogram)	10	X-ray dept.	shape of uterus — double/ septum fibroids tubes patent
laparoscopy	second half of cycle	doctor (general anaesthetic)	condition of tubes endometriosis
physical examination	any time	doctor	check general condition of uterus, vagina, ovaries

- HSG* should be postponed if there is
  - tenderness on pelvic examination
  - increasing pain on sexual intercourse
  - bad vaginal discharge
  - high risk of inflammation

or there has been an attack of salpingitis in the past three months.

OTHER TESTS SOMETIMES PERFORMED INCLUDE:

- **Testing the levels of the following hormones** to pinpoint ovulation: oestrogen, luteinizing hormone and follicle stimulating hormone. These are usually done on women whose ovarian problems have not been diagnosed by other methods.

- **Ultrasound** which can be used to detect ovulation and certain uterine problems. The interpretation is very specialized and many hospitals do not have the right staff or equipment.

- **Ovarian biopsy** which may be performed to see if there are eggs present.

- **Dilation and Curettage** which can be used to detect uterine problems such as fibroids or polyps.

- **Hysteroscopy** (inspection of uterine cavity with a telescope) which is useful for seeing any abnormalities in shape of the uterus.

- **Ferning** which is to see if the hormones are normal after ovulation. A small drop of mucus is placed on a glass slide and allowed to dry. It should crystallize into branches which look like fern leaves.

MENOPAUSE

The menopause denotes the permanent cessation of menstruation. It usually happens around the age of 50, but each woman is different. It is rare for periods to continue after the age of 55. If they do some doctors recommend an investigation because the periods may increase the risk of cancer of the womb. Menopause is also induced as a result of the removal of the ovaries — usually performed at the same time as a hysterectomy (removal of uterus).

Although around 20 to 30% of women have no discomfort during the menopause, the majority experience the characteristic symptoms of hot flushes or flashes, sweating and palpitations, high blood pressure, weight gain and distension, vaginal dryness and osteoporosis (thinning of the bones).

It is therefore common sense to arrange for your doctor to give you a medical check up around menopause. This should include:

- checking your height, weight, blood pressure,

- breast and pelvic examination,

- urine test for sugar and protein,

- blood test for anaemia,

- cervical smear,

- a discussion of any problems or symptoms that are bothering you.

The information from this check up will provide useful data if you are ill at some time in the future. Not all aches and pains or health problems are an inevitable consequence of going through the menopause and you should check any problems with your doctor. It is also recommended that women over 50 should have clinical breast examinations and regular mammography (see pp 202-4).

Women who receive oestrogen therapy after the menopause, particularly those at a higher risk of developing uterine cancer (those who are obese, diabetic or have never had children) are often offered an endometrial biopsy as a screening test.

CONCLUSION

Screening programmes have been set up in this country for a number of conditions specific to women. Their implementation has been fraught with difficulties, but the results from other countries where programmes have been successfully implemented, suggest that they should not be scrapped, but improved. The activities of pressure groups, and the media have highlighted the problems and action is now being taken to improve the service provided.

Some techniques used in the diagnosis of female complaints carry with them quite large risks and potential side effects. It is therefore important that women discuss all investigations prior to consenting to them, and establishing whether there is a less invasive alternative.

Chapter 7

MEN

Diseases which are specific to men are far fewer than those for women. This is clearly shown by the fact that there are no hospital departments which exist solely for the treatment of conditions in men, whereas all hospitals have a gynaecology department. Nevertheless some of the diseases affecting men and the male organs are serious, life threatening, and occur at a relatively young age.

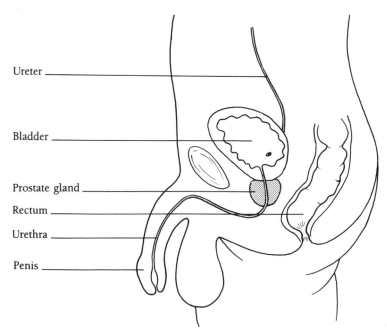

Figure 23. Sagittal section showing the male organs.

Tests for male diseases are best considered in three groups relating to the anatomy:

- the penis.

- the testicles and epididymis (the collecting tube around the testicle).

- the prostate gland.

Diseases affecting the testicle and epididymis are most common during the sexually active years. Furthermore cancer of the testicle (see below) is one of the most common cancers in men under the age of thirty and one of the most serious. Diseases of the prostate normally present in later life, though prostatic infections, particularly associated with venereal disease can occur in middle age and youth. Penile disease also occurs in the young, but more serious conditions of the penis predominate in middle to old age.

DISEASES OF THE PENIS

The majority of diseases of the penis do not require any investigation as clinical examination is usually sufficient to reveal the cause. The common conditions which occur are:

Phimosis: This is a condition where the foreskin of the penis is too tight to allow full retraction over the head of the penis. As this can result in recurrent balanitis (infection of the glans — or head — of the penis) circumcision is usually recommended. Recurrent balanitis is identified by culture of swabs taken from under the foreskin.

Paraphimosis: This occurs when the foreskin retracts but will not come back over the glans. This condition, as with phimosis, is mainly seen in children and young men. If the restriction is sufficient then reduction of blood to the glans can result and surgical treatment is usually necessary as an emergency.

Cancer of the penis: This condition is usually seen in elderly men, and starts with enlargement or a discharge. The diagnosis can only be confirmed by biopsy (see Chapter 2).

IMPOTENCE

Most male impotence (inability to achieve and sustain an erection) is thought to be of a psychological nature, but in a substantial number of patients the problem has a physical basis or may be caused by certain drugs. These drugs include:

- Alcohol (this tends to cause loss of libido rather than frank impotence)

- Guanethidine (Ismelin), methyldopa, clonidine, reserpins, propranolol, aldactone and thiazide diuretics. (All these drugs are used for treating blood pressure)

- The benzodiazepines and minor tranquillisers (e.g. librium, valium etc.)

- Antidepressants and lithium

- Anticholinergic drugs (for treating irritable bowel)

- Certain antibiotics and parasite killing drugs

- Most narcotics, marijuana and methadone

A normal male will experience penile erections during sleep, and the ability to do this is a fairly reliable indication that any complaint of impotence is psychologically caused. So a demonstration that nocturnal erections still occur can be an indication of a normal erection mechanism and as such can show to patients who consider themselves to be impotent that no physical problem exists.

TESTS FOR IMPOTENCE

Various devices are available which detect and record erection of a penis in the night. These are small electronic machines attached to rings around the penis and to a graph which charts the number, size and duration of any erections which occur during the night.

DISEASES OF THE TESTICLE AND EPIDIDYMIS

Cysts of the testicle and epididymis: These are relatively common, and appear as small pea sized or smaller swellings within the epidiymis at the lower end of the testicle. They are usually mobile, translucent (a light will shine through them as they are mainly composed of fluid) and relatively harmless. In older men a hydroele may develop which can grow to considerable size. This is a cyst, filled with fluid arising from the epididymis and which may require drainage.

Testicular torsion: The testicle is supported and supplied with blood via the spermatic cord. As well as blood vessels the cord contains muscles and a tube called the vas deferens for transporting the sperm. The cord passes from the groin into the upper part of the scrotum and thence to the testicles. The testicles are therefore suspended by the spermatic cord.

Occasionally the testicle will turn on this support producing a twist of the spermatic cord. This will cut off the blood supply to the testicle, and early diagnosis and treatment will prevent irreversible damage and subsequent loss of that testicle. Unfortunately this is a condition mainly affecting teenagers and young men, and may mimic in appearance an acute infection of the testicle and epididymis thus making early treatment difficult.

Acute epididymo-orchitis: This is an inflammatory condition of the epididymis and testicle usually caused as a complication to a viral illness, although it may result from a bacterial infection. Appropriate treatment of the superseding viral illness or antibiotic medication will resolve the condition.

Cancer of the testicles: This normally presents in men in their twenties or thirties as a enlargement of one testicle. There may be associated swelling of the inguinal glands. Urgent biopsy (See

Chapter 2) is essential in view of the serious nature of this disease. Unfortunately most cancers of the testicles are highly malignant and by the time surgery is undertaken spread of the condition has occurred.

TESTS FOR THE FUNCTION OF THE TESTICLES

The function of the testicles is twofold; the production of sperm, and the production of hormone (testosterone). Tests for these two functions are independent.

FERTILITY TESTS

Examination of the semen is the single most important test of testicular function. In infertile couples approximately 30% of the husbands prove to be infertile, and more than half can be helped by medical means. As well as spermatozoa from the testicles, the normal semen contains secretions from the prostate, some hormones, red and white blood cells, and sperm nutrients.

Tests performed on semen include examination for volume, thickness (viscosity), acidity, motility (that is the activity of the sperm), the morphology (structure of the sperm), and the amount of sperm (the number present). In addition sometimes the fructose level is assessed as this can be an indication of hormone deficiency.

A single examination of semen is not usually adequate as it takes ten weeks for sperm to form. Therefore if an abnormality is discovered, usually two further samples are necessary.

A specimen is collected after a period of sexual avoidance by either masturbation or by use of a sheath during intercourse. Some sheaths, however, contain a spermicide which chemically affects the sperm and will affect the motility count. Occasionally a more detailed test regarding fertility is performed — the post coital test, where a smear is taken from the woman's cervix after intercourse in order to assess the ability of the sperm to penetrate cervical mucus. A different cause of infertility can be the presence of sperm antibodies in the semen, which are auto antibodies made by the body, and which will damage the sperm. These antibodies can be separately identified.

NORMAL VALUES FOR SEMEN ANALYSIS

The normal values for a sperm count are:

- Volume — between 2.5 and 5mls.

- Viscosity (thickness). The specimen should be sticky at the time of collection, but become much more liquid after 15 to 30 minutes.

- Acidity — should be slightly alkaline, with a pH of 7.2 to 8.

- At least 70% of the sperm, and preferably 90% should be active (moving when seen under a microscope) for the first hour, and 50% should still be moving ten hours later.

- 80-90% of the sperm should have a normal form.

- The number of sperm present should be 60-120,000,000 per millilitre. A count below 60,000,000 per millilitre is abnormal and may be the result of organic diseases of the genitals.

An abnormality of one of these factors in the analysis may indicate where the problem lies and so aid treatment. Semen analysis is routinely carried out after vasectomy to ensure the operation has been successful. No sperm should be present.

MALE HORMONE ANALYSIS

The testicles are the main site for the production of the male hormone, testosterone, although small amounts are produced by the liver and the adrenal glands. Estimation of the blood testosterone level will give a fairly accurate indication of the function of the testicle, but may be normal when the other function of the testicle (production of sperm) is abnormal.

Until recently the urine was examined to check for adequate testicle functioning. Waste products of testosterone are chemicals known as 17-ketosteroids, and the amount of these passed over 24 hours in the urine was thought to reflect the level of production of testosterone. But this test is not totally accurate as 17-ketosteroids are also produced by the adrenal glands. One hormone excreted in the urine — Human Chorionic Gonadotrophin or HCG — can be measured and is an accurate indicator of hormone production by the testicle.

BIOPSY OF THE TESTICLE

When the analysis of the semen is abnormal, it may be necessary to check whether sperm is actually being produced in the testicle and if there is some fault with the collecting or transporting system such as a blockage. Under an anaesthetic a small section of the testicle can be removed and examined under the microscope to see whether production is adequate.

DISEASES OF THE PROSTATE

Acute prostatitis: Inflammation of the prostate gland is normally associated with gonorrhoea, other venereal diseases or following a surgical intervention such as cystoscopy. The disease causes pain in the perineum (behind the scrotum) sometimes frequency of passing water and pain on opening the bowels. If the prostatitis is very severe then complete blockage of passage of urine may occur.

Diagnosis rests on culture (see Chapter 2) of any discharge or of prostatic fluid which may be obtained by prostatic massage. Appropriate antibiotic therapy following this investigation resolves an acute infection.

Chronic prostatitis: This often follows an attack of urethritis or inflammation of the urethra. The symptoms are mainly a low grade aching pain in the perineum with frequent passage of water, and occasionally recurrent infection in the water. There may be a slight discharge from the tip of the penis and the condition may be caused by a bacterial infection or may be sterile. Bacterial identification can again be obtained by culture and microscopy of the discharge, but occasionally no culture is positive and the disease is due to sterile inflammation. In these cases the condition is extremely resistent to treatment and may persist for a long time.

Prostatic calculi (stones): In association with chronic prostatitis, small stones may form in the follicles of the gland of the prostate. This does not usually cause symptoms, but causes continuation of a chronic prostatitis.

Benign enlargement of the prostate gland: The cause of the enlargement, in later life, of the prostate gland is not known. This occurs in a very large proportion of men over sixty, and gives rise to symptoms mainly associated with urination. The urine passes from the bladder through the prostate gland, and as the gland enlarges, the drainage from the bladder becomes obstructed and this causes the first symptoms. There is difficulty with passing water, in that there is a slow start to the act of micturition, and a poor stream. Frequency of passing water also occurs and the patient often has to get up several times at night.

If the enlargement continues sufficiently and the obstruction is further increased then the bladder and the kidneys will be affected.

The diagnosis is mainly based on examination, but cytoscopy (see Chapter 2) will disclose the enlargement.

Cancer of the prostate: Cancer of the prostate occurs mainly in older men, but as the symptoms are similar to benign obstruction they may be overlooked. Occasionally it occurs at a younger age, and consequently symptoms of obstruction in middle life may create greater concern as cancer is more likely. Sometimes cancer of the prostate can cause no symptoms, and only be found when removed at excision of the gland. Cancer is the cause of the obstruction in about 20% of patients suffering from prostate disease. The symptoms of prostate cancer are similar to those of benign hypertrophy as enlargement of the gland occurs initially. Examination may also be similar, but often enlargement is more irregular.

TESTS OF THE FUNCTION OF THE PROSTATE

In suspected prostatic disease microscopy and culture of the urine and the prostatic fluid should be performed, and if necessary an intravenous pyelogram to show any abnormality within the kidneys. Blood tests may be performed to estimate the blood urea (an estimate of kidney function) and the serum acid phosphatese (see below). Normally in addition cystoscopy is carried out immediately prior to operation, or before, if there is some doubt in the diagnosis.

TESTS FOR CANCER OF THE PROSTATE

Prostatic biopsy: In this test a hollow needle is inserted via the rectum into the prostate gland. A core of tissue is thus removed in the centre of the needle which is then examined under the microscope. Cancer may be shown in the specimens.

Serum acid phosphatase: The prostate gland produces acid phosphatase and discharges a proportion into the blood. In cancer of the prostate, an excessive amount is produced and causes high levels of acid phosphatase in the blood. A raised level of acid phosphatase is therefore diagnostic of cancer of the prostate.

A recent test for the presence of sperm in forensic medicine is the demonstration of prostatic acid phosphatase secreted by the prostate gland during intercourse in the vagina in rape cases or on clothing.

SELF EXAMINATION IN MEN

Self examination of the breasts in women is recommended for the early detection of breast cancer. In view of the serious consequences of late diagnosis of cancer of the testicles in men, self examination in them is probably of equal importance.

The tests should be performed in a relaxed and warm environment, and should take the following form:

Standing naked in front of a full length mirror, observe whether there is any apparent difference in the size, texture of the skin or position of the testicles. (It is normal for one testicle to be slightly higher than the other, but this situation should not change). Then carefully feel each testicle, trying to note whether there is any irregular enlargement, swelling or lumps, either on the surface of the testicle or within the surrounding tissue. Lumps which are quite separate from the testicle are usually in the epididymis (the collecting tubes at the base of the testicle) and are usually harmless, but any swelling or lumps on the testicle itself demand early investigation. This may include an exploration of the testicle surgically with a biopsy. Despite this, in view of the rapid spread of so many cancers of the testicle, diagnostic accuracy is vital in order to ensure adequate and early treatment.

Chapter 8

MENTAL HEALTH

Mental health is perhaps one of the most controversial areas of medicine. Certainly we fear the diseases of the mind — striking as they do, at the core of being human — the personality, the way we relate to one another, think and talk. And once labelled as mentally ill the consequences to the individual can be enormous — loss of jobs, driving licence, family and friends.

Psychiatry — the branch of medicine that deals with mental health — with its draconian past of Bedlam and chains, does little to allay those fears. Its peculiar relationship to the law makes one feel that psychiatrists can — even if they rarely do — enforce their diagnosis and treatment against the wishes of their patients. Psychiatrists are traditionally custodians — with a greater emphasis on protecting society from the mental sick, rather than treating those they have removed from society.

While it is clear that psychiatry has moved on from a merely custodial role, there is still considerable dispute about the classification, diagnosis, prognosis and treatment of mental disorders. It is difficult, therefore, to provide a simple outline of the testing within psychiatry. Instead, this chapter is an overview, rather than a detailed list.

CLASSIFICATION

Classification in any discipline, is an important guide to diagnosis and treatment. In psychiatry, classification is based mainly on descriptions of symptoms, signs and the course of the disorders, as so little is known about the cause of mental disorders. Broadly speaking there are seven categories of mental disorders:

- those thought to be due to a malfunction of the brain, such as senility

- those thought to be due to severe mental illness, such as schizophrenia, severe depression and mania

- those attributable to reactions to stress, such as anxiety states and phobias, hysterical states, obsessive compulsive states and milder depression

- those relating to the development of the personality; this category includes mental handicap — intellectual and emotional, and immaturities of personality

- those where bodily changes are significantly related to emotional factors, ie psychosomatic disorders

- sexual disorders

- alcoholism and drug abuse

CAUSES OF MENTAL ILLNESS

In the past, mental illness was often viewed as a punishment from God or as evidence of an individual having consorted with the devil. Today there is still an aura of guilt and moral responsibility associated with mental illness. There is a suspicion that a person who is mentally ill must have brought his problems on himself and that he could cure himself if he would just 'pull himself together'.

The actual causes of mental illness remain elusive. So far implicated are:

- brain abnormalities

- heredity

- environmental factors including viral infection, abnormalities in the nourishment the brain receives, head injuries, as well as the stresses of everyday life.

APPROACHES TO PSYCHIATRY

Psychiatry has developed in a number of different directions in the last hundred years. Some psychiatrists have taken a psychoanalytic and psychodynamic approach — as developed by Freud and his followers. This approach looks at the interplay of the unconscious, the preconscious, and the conscious in the functioning of the human mind. Other psychiatrists took a more empirical approach, either studying — like the American psychologist B.F. Skinner — human behaviour not the mind in order to understand mental health; or taking a biological approach like Emil Kraepelin, whose classification of mental disease has remained in use for nearly a hundred years. He developed the concepts of manic-depressive insanity and dementia praecox (schizophrenia). In addition to these two major illnesses, he described several others, such as psychoses occurring in late life (paraphrenia) and disorders characterized primarily by delusional thinking with relative preservation of other functions.

As other branches of medicine have become more scientific and specialized, so psychiatrists strived for a firmer pathological basis to their theories in order to achieve equal status. This has sometimes led to artificial extensions of categories of illness. And, with the development of new drug therapies which can reduce or even eliminate symptoms of major illnesses like schizophrenia or depression, psychiatrists have concentrated more and more on the biological approach — sometimes at the expense of the more emotionally based aspects of mental health. There is however, a tendency to give patients with emotional disturbances a hard psychiatric label to justify the use of a psychotropic drug. Since these drugs are illness specific there is a risk, if inaccurate diagnoses are being made, that the patient will get worse, not better as a result of taking the drugs.

THREE MODELS OF MENTAL ILLNESS

	Psychodynamic	Behavioural	Biological
Emphasis	Mind	Behaviour	Brain

	Psychodynamic	Behavioural	Biological
Causes of illness	(i) Disturbed dynamics (ii) Childhood experiences	Learned habits	Biological imbalances
Methods of study	Introspection (free association dream analysis)	Controlled experiences (use of conditioning, animal research)	Neuro-sciences (neuro-chemistry, behavioural genetics)
Types of illness	Mild (neuroses, personality disorders)	Mild to severe (neuroses, personality disorders, addictions)	Moderate to severe (depression, mania, schizo-phrenia)
Method of treatment	Psychotherapy	Behaviour modification	Medication

(from *The Broken Brain: The biological revolution in Psychiatry* by Nancy C. Andreasen, 1984 NY: Harper & Row)

PSYCHIATRY AND THE LAW

There is special relationship between Psychiatry and the law that does not exist in other branch of medicine. The law requires an individual to be of 'sound mind' before s/he can enter any legal contract — such as a marriage, or stand trial for a crime. Insanity though, like guilt must be proved which is where the psychiatrists become involved. It is, however, the law that defines the terms and is the final arbiter in all interpretations of medico-legal problems. The other side of this relationship with the law deals with the problem that mentally ill people are sometimes unable to recognize that they need help, so therefore help may have to be imposed on them. This is dealt with in Section 2 of the Mental

Health Act (1983) under 'compulsory admission' (see on).

According to the Mental Health Act, 'mental disorders' are divided into four categories:

Mental Impairment: 'a state of arrested or incomplete development of mind which includes significant impairment of intelligence and social functioning and is associated with abnormally aggressive or seriously irresponsible conduct on the part of the person concerned'.

Severe Mental Impairment: 'a state of arrested or incomplete development of mind which includes severe impairment of intelligence and social functioning and is associated with abnormally aggressive or seriously irresponsible conduct on the part of the person concerned'.

Psychopathic Disorder: 'a persistent disorder or disability of mind (whether or not including significant impairment of intelligence) which results in abnormally aggressive or seriously irresponsible conduct on the part of the person concerned'. Promiscuity, immoral conduct, sexual deviancy or dependence on alcohol or drugs are not included.

Mental Illness: as yet there is no statutory definition of this category; it is taken to be that which is professionally accepted at the time.

These categories are extraordinarily vague. There seems to be some implicit definition of normality from which the categories are derived. But what is normality or non-conformity? Where does eccentricity end and a mental disorder begin? What is deviation, and from what? How do you judge someone to have a 'significant impairment of intelligence?' And when is seriously irresponsible or aggressive behaviour madness, and when is it merely anti-social behaviour?

Psychiatry, because it deals with intangibles like delusions, and cannot agree on diagnosis, provides treatments that have been introduced on insufficient evidence, and when its relationships with the law are so vague and contentious, is open to manipulation both from within and without. There is always the danger of the law on mental health being abused for political or financial gain.

We have already seen in the USSR, for example, psychiatrists diagnose schizophrenia in dissidents on the basis of 'reformist delusions'.

COMPULSORY ADMISSION

Compulsory admission into hospital for assessment and/or treatment requires two medical recommendations — one from a psychiatrist (approved by the Health Authority), and one from another registered medical practitioner — preferably one who knows the patient, such as his or her GP. The doctors must examine the individual within five days of each other, and then an application for admission is needed by an approved social worker or the nearest relative. Once all documentation is complete the individual can be admitted for 28 days. He or she can appeal to a Mental Health Review Tribunal in the first 14 days. The responsible doctor in the hospital can also discharge the patient home if appropriate, or can cancel the order so that the patient remains informally. The nearest relative can also discharge the patient. In an emergency an individual can be admitted with a recommendation from any one doctor and an application by a social worker or the nearest relative — admission must then be within 24 hours, and holds for 72 hours, until the fuller procedure can be invoked.

Compulsory admission for treatment can be for up to six months; and, since this is a more serious infringement of civil rights there are additional safeguards. The medical recommendations have to be filled in with more detail of the evidence for the diagnosis, and must state that the treatment is necessary for the health and safety of the patient or for the protection of other persons, and cannot be provided unless the patient is detained. The patients on treatment orders can be discharged early by their nearest relative, the responsible medical officer, the administering Heath Authority of the hospital or a Mental Health Review Tribunal, to which the patient has a right of direct appeal.

However, the majority (around 95%) of psychiatric patients in hospitals are there of their own free will. People seeking psychiatric help have the same legal rights as other citizens who consult doctors. Referral to a psychiatrist occurs in exactly the same way as referral to any medical specialist and most patients will be completely unaffected by the Mental Health Act.

VISITING A PSYCHIATRIST

Diagnosis of most psychiatric conditions is essentially a judgement made by the psychiatrist, since laboratory investigations are only helpful in the minority of cases and most assessments are made on the basis of extensive interviews.

THE INTERVIEW

During an interview with a psychiatrist you will be asked to describe what your problems are in your own words. He or she will then ask you questions about your illness or disorder, such as:

- how long it has been going on

- symptoms, including changes in sleep, appetite, mood, energy, and concentration

- what might have precipitated it

- the effect of the illness on personal relationships and working efficiency

- treatment so far.

After establishing the history of your illness the psychiatrist will want to know about your family and personal history.

Family History: The doctor will want to know your parents and any siblings ages, occupations, health — including any family history of psychiatric illnesses or alcoholism. If any of these relatives are dead, then the doctor will ask for the date, cause of death and your age at the time. The doctor may cast his or her net wider, asking about cousins, aunts, grandparents and so on. This will almost certainly be the case if there is the possibility of a strong genetic factor being involved in the suspected disorder.

Personal History: You will be asked to provide quite a detailed account of your life history, from infancy to the present day. This will include information on:

- any complications during pregnancy or birth, serious illnesses in infancy, or delays in development

- your home environment: place of birth, other places of residence, the relationship you had with those you grew up with and important events in your childhood

- your schooling: academic achievements, your relationships with other children, and your attitude to teachers

- any 'neurotic traits' such as nail-biting, bed-wetting, although their presence does not predict adult neurosis

- your work: what jobs you have had, success and satisfaction associated with them and reasons for change

- your sexual life: this will only be explored if it is relevant to the present complaint

- your marital history: duration of marriage, spouse's age, occupation, health and your relationship with them. Information will be required about any previous marriages and reasons for their ending

- your children: their names, ages, health, your relationship with them

- your medical history: past illnesses, present physical symptoms, treatment

- your past psychiatric history: dates of previous episodes of illness, diagnosis, treatment

- your present circumstances: type of accommodation, people in household, financial or practical problems.

The doctor will also make an assessment of your premorbid personality — ie your personality before the onset of the presenting complaint. This will include an estimation of:

- your ability to make friends and relate to those in authority

- your mood: for example, cheerful, or despondent, anxious or placid, tendency to mood swings, outbursts of temper, response to stress

- your character: for example, confident or diffident, independent or reliant on others, conscientious and perfectionist

- your levels of energy and activity

- your attitudes to religion, politics, membership of groups or societies, hobbies

- alcohol and tobacco consumption, drug abuse

- criminal behaviour

An extremely important part of a psychiatrist's repertoire for assessing a patient is an *examination of mental state.* Observations will be made on:

- general appearance and behaviour

- talk: manner and content

- subjective state: mood and attitude to the consultation

- content of thought including disorders of thinking, obsessive-compulsive phenomena, ideas of reference and delusions and other pre-occupying themes

- contact with reality — delusion, hallucinations and illusions

- cognition and intelligence: including

  - memory: long-term memory is assessed from the history taking. Tests of short-term memory include the ability to repeat a name and address both immediately and after five minutes and the number of digits a patient is able to repeat back to the interviewer

  - orientation: in time (day, date, time of day), in place, and in person (by identification of the interviewer or ward staff)

  - attention and concentration: tests include ability to list the months of the year in reverse order, and subtraction of serial sevens from 100, ie 93, 86, 79, and so on

  - general information: the psychiatrist will ask questions appropriate to your educational level. Average questions include the name of the Monarch, Prime Minister, and the names of six large towns

  - intelligence as estimated by the interviewer

  - your insight and judgement, for example, of your illness

There are a wide variety of tests that have been introduced to assess mental state. Which, if any test will be used in any one interview depends on the orientation and training of the examining psychiatrists.

PHYSICAL EXAMINATION

If you are an in-patient, then you will almost certainly have a physical examination, including a neurological one. Ideally out-patients should have one too, but in practice only people in whom there is reason to suspect an organic cause to the disorder will have one.

INTERVIEW WITH INFORMANT

Psychiatrists will on occasion — usually if an individual is too disturbed or uncooperative to give a full history — arrange a separate interview with an 'informant' — a member of the individual's close family or a work colleague, for example. However this should only be done with the patient's consent. These interviews are particularly important in establishing the individual's premorbid personality.

After completing the above procedures, the doctor will formulate a critical summary of the case which will include; suggestions of diagnosis with evidence for and against; intended further investigations such as a social worker's report, psychological testing and laboratory tests; the plan for management, and comments on prognosis.

FURTHER INVESTIGATIONS

Laboratory tests: There are laboratory tests that may help illuminate the physical processing underlying the patient's symptoms.

Brain imaging: e.g. CT scans, nuclear magnetic imaging, positron-emission tomographic scanning. Brain imaging can detect certain types of schizophrenia and dementia because there are common abnormalities in the brain.

Neurochemical tests: samples of blood and urine are studied to determine whether they contain unusually large or small amounts of chemicals known to occur in the brain or known to affect people's emotional and mental condition.

Measurement of brain waves — EEG: electrodes are placed on the scalp using a salty jelly that aids the transmission of electrical impulses. The electrodes are attached by wire to a recording device. We know quite a bit about the patterns of brain waves that tend to occur in normal people when awake and asleep so a patient's EEG can be compared with these patterns. EEG only provides a crude measure of brain function and until relatively recently, its chief application in psychiatry has been to rule out various neurological diseases that may masquerade as psychiatric disease. Researchers have found that the clinically depressed have abnormal EEG patterns during sleep which implies that something has gone wrong with the brain's regulatory mechanisms from depression. This ties in with the fact that many depressives are also insomniacs.

Psychological tests: There are an enormous number of such tests although they are seldom enough on their own to diagnose organic impairment which is not clinically obvious, but they can provide evidence for or against its presence in doubtful cases. They are helpful in assessing the severity and location of the impairment in known cases, and repeated testing can be useful in monitoring progress. Tests used include those of intelligence, memory perception, and ability for abstract thinking.

MENTAL ABILITY

Another aspect of mental health is the assessment of mental ability. This has been attempted through

- intelligence tests

- achievement tests

- aptitude tests

- personality tests

There is no real standardization for any of these and all are open to interpretation. However, we are all at some point subjected to them — at school, for jobs and so on. What is known is that the more you take the tests the easier you find them — so practice is a good idea.

CONCLUSIONS

Testing for mental health is still a very crude science. The individuals on whom the tests are employed are often not — by the nature of their disorder — in a position to question the tests' validity or value. And not everybody has friends or relatives who will ensure the medical help being provided is in their best interests. However, psychiatry has come a long way in the past ten years and is continuing to change. With greater understanding of the nature of mental disorders will come improvements in the methods used to diagnose them.

Chapter 9

CONCLUSION

We have been struck while writing this book by the importance of good history taking and thorough physical examination in the assessment of a patient. Medical testing is not an alternative to such an assessment — only an adjunct. Unfortunately doctors have been well and truly confused by the technological revolution, and like their patients they are ready to believe that machinery, rather than humans, must be better equipped to actually pinpoint patients' problems. The machine is only as good as its maker — and its user, and therein lies a problem. Too often a test is introduced without proper evaluation, and then operated by insufficiently trained technicians. Furthermore, ever increasing demands and expectations from patients allow less and less time for the doctor to make a thorough examination. In a hard pressed surgery after a busy day, a doctor may be tempted to perform another test on a patient which means quickly filling in a form rather than conducting yet another examination. Unfortunately such an approach is often counter-productive in that it frequently provides a negative and therefore useless test, fails to resolve the patient's problem, and leads to increasingly greater demands from the patient in terms of more and more tests. Furthermore there is a trend towards over testing, merely because the tests are there. As a result a physician can be faced with too much information — often conflicting — from which to make his assessment.

Nobody would suggest that high technology medical testing is entirely a bad thing. Clearly such techniques as CT scans and MNR imaging have significantly improved the ability of the doctors to diagnose previously difficult conditions. But what is also clear — even to the medical profession — is that this technology is not used effectively enough — the rate of mis-diagnosis is alarmingly high — up to 15%. If medical tests are to be performed, it is imperative that certain criteria should be met.

For example:

1. The medical test should be tested. Is it safe? Is it accurate? Is it cost effective? Does it improve on tests currently available, or add to information already in the possession of the doctor? These questions must be adequately answered before introducing a new test.

2. Once a test has been evaluated and approved, the technicians performing the test need to be thoroughly trained in its use, and all personnel handling the results must be trained in their interpretation.

3. Interpretation of results should be standardized throughout the country and between countries — preferably in line with the rest of Europe and America. This would reduce the confusion that can result when an individual moves from one health authority or country to another.

4. If a test has been shown to be valuable and safe, it should then be available to all who need it. Less safe or accurate tests should be recalled from hospitals and clinics.

5. Doctors should always assess whether the test is really necessary before they perform it, or order it. The procedures should then be explained to the patient and the doctor should discuss the risks and benefits involved. Only then will the patient be in a position to make an informed decision as to whether or not to agree to the test.

Future trends in medical testing are difficult to predict. The crystal ball is clouded by political and financial issues. While various political parties differ widely on how health care should be provided in this country, the present administration seems set on a course that could eventually destroy the National Health Service as we know it — and perhaps the whole Welfare State. It seems keen to mimic America, with private medicine being the norm and 'free' medical care being available in only exceptional circumstances. How this would work in Britain is hard to assess. At the moment we all pay very high National Insurance contributions which are supposed, amongst other things, to pay for our health care. It is difficult to see how people are going to be able to find the extra cash for private insurance in addition to these yearly payments. The Government does not seem willing to reduce or abolish NI contributions — presumably because of the additional revenue it represents. Until the details become clear as to how health care is going to change, we can only surmise on the fate of medical testing.

In the next few years things are unlikely to change, although with an increase in patients and a decrease in resources, doctors may be forced to rationalize the testing they perform. Certainly a lot of money could be saved if testing was rationalized — releasing it for other aspects of health care.

Doctors, particularly pathologists, are worried about the high rates of mis-diagnosis. Up to 15% of patients who die in hospital are found, on post mortem, to have been mis-diagnosed in a 'clinically significant' way.

A few hospitals have responded to the challenge this statistic represents. For example, in Nottingham, the staff — doctors, nurses, radiographers, technicians and students — at the General Hospital meet regularly to discuss the diagnosis of patients. At Northwick Park Hospital in London, they have implemented a system whereby radiographers mark X-rays they think indicate a problem. This alerts the Casualty Officers, who in the past had been missing many problems clearly indicated on the X-ray. Unfortunately, too many hospitals are gripped by a lethargy which prevents them from implementing such simple innovations. We can only hope in the future that more hospitals will throw off this malaise and seek ways of reducing their rates of mis-diagnosis.

It would be foolish to consider that our present knowledge of human physiology and anatomy is complete. It may well be that future years will see methods of diagnosis which at the moment are entirely unknown. Medicine had progressed throughout the last few hundred years at ever increasing rates, and there is no reason to consider that this should end. For example there may be a physiological system beneath that which is at present understood. There do seem to be electro-magnetic changes within cells that precede cellular changes caused by disease. It is conceivable that diagnosis at this energetic level could produce much earlier diagnosis of clinical problems, and therefore even earlier potential treatment.

In addition it is possible that our present ideas regarding the causation of disease might change. Many conditions at the moment are considered to be viral in origin but this may not always be the case. Increasingly we are becoming aware of environment factors which can influence our health, such as pollution, radiation, and allergies, and it may well be that these and other encounters in our every-day lives may eventually be accepted as causative.

An innovation the authors would like to see is an increase in preventative medicine — with the emphasis on actively maintaining the health of the population rather than waiting until people fall sick before acting. Regular health check-ups should be encouraged, in conjunction with advice on exercise and healthy diets. Screening is also a potentially powerful tool in health care — if properly implemented. Badly implemented it is worse than useless. There needs to be an improvement in our screening programmes in this country, identifying — where possible — 'at risk' groups. This would catch diseases early and avoid the necessity of invasive and dangerous treatments.

Change is possible. We have seen food manufacturers bow to informed consumer pressure — labelling food and providing healthy less processed products. To improve medical testing in this country, the public again needs to be informed — and we hope this book will go some way towards achieving that goal.

INDEX

INDEX